Home Birth

Why do women choose to give birth at home, even in situations defined as medically risky? Are they ignorant? Irresponsible? Risking their babies' lives for their own good experience? Mary L. Nolan explores this uncharted territory with respect and intelligence, creating a fascinating and invaluable resource for carers involved with home birth and/or women with 'high risk' pregnancies. Women and families choosing home birth will especially enjoy the voices of strong-minded women who are making their own choices.

Dr Sarah J. Buckley, author, *Gentle Birth, Gentle Mothering*
www.sarahjbuckley.com

This is a book for midwives, midwifery students and all those various health professionals who work with pregnant women but it is one which starts from women's stories and their points of view. It links women's lived experience directly to midwifery best practice in relation to home birth.

Home Birth tells ten women's stories, focusing on the ways in which the women were helped or hindered, supported or deterred during their journey towards a home birth. It will describe the actual births through the eyes of the women, and the first few hours afterwards. Providing an understanding of how best to meet women's physical, psychological, social and spiritual needs in childbirth, the text examines how women perceive and experience professional concerns relating to the safety of home birth in particular circumstances, such as following caesarean section; when the mother is a teenager or over 40; or when she has a pre-existing medical condition.

Pointers to best practice are presented succinctly alongside the narratives of women's pregnancies and births, making this a practical and relevant read for all those concerned with making home birth a real option for women.

Mary L. Nolan is Professor of Perinatal Education at the University of Worcester, UK. She is also Senior Tutor at the National Childbirth Trust.

Home Birth
The politics of difficult choices

Mary L. Nolan

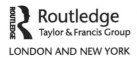

Routledge
Taylor & Francis Group

LONDON AND NEW YORK

First published 2011
by Routledge
2 Park Square, Milton Park, Abingdon, Oxon, OX14 4RN

Simultaneously published in the USA and Canada
by Routledge
711 Third Avenue, New York, NY 10017

*Routledge is an imprint of the Taylor & Francis Group,
an informa business*

© 2011 Mary L. Nolan

Typeset in Sabon by
Pindar NZ, Auckland, New Zealand

British Library Cataloguing in Publication Data
A catalogue record for this book is available from the British Library

Library of Congress Cataloging-in-Publication Data
Nolan, Mary, 1956–
Home birth : the politics of difficult choices / Mary L. Nolan.
    p. ; cm.
  Includes bibliographical references.
  1. Childbirth at home—Great Britain—Decision making. I. Title.
  [DNLM: 1. Home Childbirth. 2. Health Policy. 3. Informed
Consent. 4. Patient Compliance. WQ 155 N788h 2011]
  RG661.5.N65 2011
  618.4—dc22   2010022493

ISBN13: 978-0-415-55754-2 (hbk)
ISBN13: 978-0-415-55755-9 (pbk)
ISBN13: 978-0-203-83667-5 (ebk)

Contents

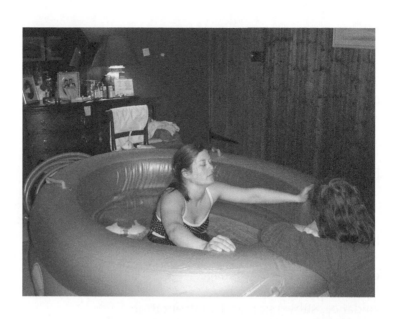

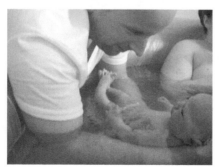
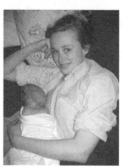

Acknowledgements

It has been such a pleasure to write this book. A pleasure because of the opportunity it gave me to meet remarkable women and men, all of whom were eager to help me, often welcoming me into their homes, and following up interviews with supportive phone calls and emails. In particular, I would like to mention the following ardent and articulate home birth mothers: Rosie, Catherine, Jo, Genevieve, Lynn, Maria, Toni, Vivien, Cher, Kirsten, Isma, Jane, Sarah, Wendy and Jean. There are fathers who should also be mentioned, and especially Will and Jonathan. I am very grateful to Emma for permission to use her wonderful home birth photo for the front cover.

The book was also dependent on long conversations with my husband, Peter, during a six weeks period spent abroad when most of the chapters were written. His unflagging support and constantly declared interest in my project (even when I am sure he was not interested!) were irreplaceable.

Finally, I would like to thank the staff at Funchal Library for making me so welcome when I arrived every day for my six hours stint in their very comfortable study room. The peaceful environment at the library, only occasionally interrupted by the delightful visits of local schoolchildren, assisted me greatly with my task.

1 Policy

Does it mean what it says?

It has been said that the happiest people in the world live in countries where they can make choices, where there is a high degree of tolerance of the choices that they make, and where the political system is one of 'government of the people, by the people, for the people' (Abraham Lincoln 1863). Based on these criteria, Denmark would apparently appear to be a very happy place to live, and the United Kingdom and America less so (www.worldvalues-survey.com).

In the UK, women have experienced democracy only since 1912, when they were finally granted the vote as a result of the heroic efforts of Emmeline Pankhurst and the Suffragettes. Prior to this, women played no part in choosing the government, and had very few choices in their personal lives. When they married, they became the property of their husbands and in the absence of contraception, had limited choice as to when and how often they became pregnant.

The women who fought for the vote were described in at least one American newspaper as engaged in 'ruffianly acts' and as initiating a 'new terrorism' (Harbor Grace Standard 24 August 1912). They knew what they wanted and why they wanted it. They were able to mount arguments that were as good as, and very often better than those of their opponents. Opponents were not only found among men; many women were also opposed to female suffrage.

Today, despite ongoing inequality in, for example, men's and women's pay, it might be considered that women have far more choices than their early twentieth-century sisters were able to make. Yet choice in maternity care remains limited because nulliparous women are unfamiliar with childbirth owing to its removal from the domestic domain, by lack of availability of alternatives to hospital as the location for birth, by the prevailing culture of fear surrounding childbirth and by professional dominance in the maternity service. In 1970, the Peel Report (DHSS) recommended that all women should have their babies in hospital. Doubtless the motivation of those who sat on the committee that drew up the Report was to protect women and babies. Nonetheless, in 1986, the decade after the Report appeared, a medical statistician called Marjorie Tew was able to demonstrate that home birth was at least as safe as hospital birth, and possibly safer. In the wake of numerous studies investigating whether Tew's analysis was right, the National Institute for Health and Clinical Excellence (NICE) concluded that:

> The change to planned hospital birth for low-risk pregnant women in many countries during this century was not supported by good evidence. Planned hospital birth may even increase unnecessary interventions and complications without any benefit for low-risk women.
>
> (Olsen and Jewell 1998)

There was little resistance to Peel, however, or challenge to the maternity service until the early 1980s, when Janet Balaskas and Sheila Kitzinger organized the 'Birthrights Rally' on Hampstead Heath in April 1982. The protest was for women to have the right to labour and give birth actively, rather than comply with an 'actively managed' birth, lying flat on their backs, legs in stirrups, surrounded by medical staff, with bright lights focussed on their genitals. Birth did begin to change, but very slowly. Women were 'allowed' to be upright for labour; delivery suites were painted in pastel colours to make the environment more user-friendly, and government policy started informing childbearing women of their 'choices'.

Real choice as to place of birth, however, remains illusory for most women, and it could be that most women don't want it. It's a step too far to choose where to have your baby. Choosing which school to send your child to, or how to pay your electricity bill, or which hospital to attend for your hip replacement are choices that have been far more readily accepted, although they are perhaps not made as freely as people imagine. Everyone's choices are restricted, as they have always been, by their temperament, educational, social and economic status, by their relationships with significant others, by religion and culture. Choice is not an even playing field; it is not free to all and it is not entirely free. As Baz Luhrmann (1998) reminded us: 'Your choices are half chance; so are everybody else's'.

Home birth is not a choice that is often chosen by women in the UK today. Women don't see it as a choice that sensible women living in a country where the best medical technologies are available would make. This is a situation with unexpected ramifications because choices made by the affluent appear to the less affluent as the best choices to make. So the choice to have your baby in hospital, a choice that is, in fact, only safe in certain parts of the world, becomes, unfortunately, the preferred choice for women from poor countries who do not have access to the kind of hospitals their rich sisters frequent. I attended a conference recently where an official of the World Health Organization described visiting a hospital in Bangladesh (Merialdi 2010). A woman who had just given birth to a premature baby lay on a filthy bed in a ward where the ambient temperature was around 40°C. At the other end of the ward was an incubator (Western style) plugged into the wall, but not functioning. The 1.2kg baby lay in the incubator where the temperature was exactly the same as that on the ward. Had the mother held the baby against her skin, she would have been able to regulate her baby's temperature far more effectively.

In Bangladesh, the maternal mortality rate is 320/100,000 and the neonatal mortality rate is 41/1000 live births (www.unfpa-bangladesh.org). Giving birth is risky. Hospitals appear to be places of safety to poor women when women with a far greater range of choices in their everyday lives choose to have their babies there. And when poor women are told that very few Western women (or women from the rich cities of China and India) choose to have their babies at home, they make the intelligent decision to go to hospital. Thus it is that privileged women need to exercise their choices around having babies so that they do not bear the responsibility for misleading women whose choices are neither so varied nor of such high quality.

Over the last 25 years, the UK National Health Service has developed a rhetoric of choice sometimes unsubstantiated by people's lived experience of health care. Nowhere has this rhetoric been so powerful or sustained as in relation to the maternity services. In 1993, *Changing Childbirth* famously described three standards upon which maternity care should be based and by which it should be judged; these were Choice, Continuity and Control. Women should be able to *choose* the pattern of care they want for themselves and their baby, including where to give birth. They should experience *continuity* of care from a small group of health professionals whom they can get to know well during the course of their pregnancies, and should thereby feel that they have *control* over what happens to them during the childbearing year.

In 2007, *Maternity Matters* (DH) reiterated the pledges of more than a decade previously and stated that choice for women should exist in four areas: choice of how to access maternity care, choice of type of antenatal care, choice of place of birth and choice of place of postnatal care. All targets are proving difficult to hit, and not least, choice of place of birth. The most recent report on the availability of home birth was published by the National Childbirth Trust (NHS) in 2009. Entitled, *Location, Location, Location*, it demonstrated how the national home birth rate of 2.7 per cent in 2007 hid considerable differences between the rates in individual local authorities where the rate varied from less than 1 per cent to more than 10 per cent.

Writing in *Maternity Matters* (2007), the Secretary of State observed that:

> Increasing choice will improve the quality and family friendliness of maternity services and encourage good services to improve even more.
>
> (p. 2)

Yet, there is a caveat. *Maternity Matters* also states:

> The national choice guarantees described in this document are . . .
>   Choice of place of birth –

Depending on their circumstances [author's emphasis], women and their partners will be able to choose between three different options. These are:

- a home birth
- birth in a local facility, including a hospital, under the care of a midwife
- birth in a hospital supported by a local maternity care team including midwives, anaesthetists and consultant obstetricians.

(p. 5)

The only clarification provided by the report of the overt caveat contained in the words 'depending on the circumstances' is that, 'for some women [hospital birth] will be the safest option' (p. 5). Perhaps there is also what might be described as a hidden persuader, a subliminal message to influence the choice of the targeted patient group without their being aware of it, in the detailed account of the support available in hospital – support consisting of three groups of health professionals. By contrast, there is no mention of any support at home; indeed there is no mention of anything being provided by the NHS at home, and even birth in 'a local facility' (a midwife-led unit or birth centre) is not described as 'supported' but rather as being 'under the care of a midwife'.

The rhetoric attempts to subtly persuade that some choices are richer than others, and perhaps, safer than others. Let me offer an example of how this works.

A mother suggests two possible day trips that she and her child might take – they can go to Sea World or to a museum. The mother would rather go to the museum because it's cheaper and there's a pleasant coffee shop where she can take a rest during the outing. The child would rather go to Sea World. The mother informs the child that there is an ice-cream shop next to the museum and a visit there is a distinct possibility. The child must now choose.

One child chooses the museum. Why? Because he knows that is where his mother would rather go and he likes to please his Mum.

Another child also chooses the museum. The attraction of ice-cream outweighs the attraction of Sea World, although the museum is not as satisfying as the main focus of the trip.

A third child chooses Sea World. His mother indicates by her body language that she is disappointed. The child is puzzled, perceiving that the 'choice' was not quite as straightforward as he had imagined. He changes his mind and opts for the museum.

A fourth child chooses Sea World. He ignores his mother's slumped body language and reckons that a choice is a choice. However, his trip is not as satisfactory as he had hoped because his mother isn't wholeheartedly out to enjoy it.

In three of these scenarios, the mother gets what she really wants. In the fourth, she doesn't, but she effectively destroys both her own and her child's enjoyment of the trip by her attitude. An ethicist might argue that none of the four scenarios represents the exercise of a free and democratic choice on the part of the child.

Much has been written in the midwifery press and in books for midwives about choice, about home birth, and about keeping women at the centre of maternity care. This book looks at the really difficult choices that women sometimes insist on making, at the choices that health care professionals feel are self-evidently misguided, and at the grey area of *Maternity Matters* (2007), which is represented by the words 'depending on their circumstances'. It examines the conflict between women's innate knowledge and institutional knowledge, and looks at what happens when public concern about the safety of babies attempts to override the knowledge that mothers have of themselves and their circumstances. The stories of ten women are told in this book. The women are unusual in that they insisted on having exactly what maternity policy claims to be offering – namely choice of type of care. Unlike many women and health care users generally, they did not accept institutional definitions of 'choice' or limitations imposed on choice by individual health care professionals, but asked for the fullness of choice as, they believed, it is enshrined in health care policy. They wanted the very best of what that policy says should be on offer. What they found was that maternity care practice was antagonistic to their expectations and aspirations, and that the service is highly selective in terms of whose choices it chooses to embrace.

The book gives priority to these ten women's stories. Who better to evaluate health care policy than the people who refuse to be constructed by it? Policy is generally successful in shaping the way in which people approach, utilize and evaluate services, but in order for it to develop and mature, it is important to examine the experiences of the people who ask why the policy seems to be offering something that those charged with delivering it are out of sympathy with or that they interpret very differently from how it appears to service users.

The book therefore accepts the primacy of the knowledge which those who use the service have of the service. In addition to quoting directly from the evidence provided by the women, it also draws on evidence from the literature of choice, midwifery and obstetrics, from the media and from anecdote. The book does not accept that knowledge is the preserve of any one of these, but is instead predicated on the assumption that all have a contribution to make to understanding what happens when policy interfaces with the service and the service interfaces with health care users.

Each chapter identifies themes from the women's experiences of care, quoting from their stories in an attempt to understand the women themselves, their motivation, their passion, their stubbornness, and how a service dedicated to their well-being presented itself to them and was interpreted by them. The book raises questions about the nature of policy and what happens when there is the potential for multiple readings of its intentions and of the way in which it should be delivered. Policy may determine the direction of health care, but those who formulate it are rarely, if ever, those who must deliver it. Those who deliver it are constrained by 'best evidence' (which in turn is dependent on the extent of the research that has been carried out and on its quality), by shortages of staff and limited budgets, by fear of bosses, litigation and birth itself, and by time. Patients may take health care policy at face value, not questioning whether there are the resources of money, time and personnel, to deliver it. The stage is set for frustration on all sides, and perhaps for actions borne out of desperation or resentment.

The situations in which the women in this book found themselves challenge the democracy of health care in the UK today, and raise worrying issues about iatrogenic stress and its potential impact on the safety of women and babies, the safety that everyone, mothers and fathers first and health care professionals next, are all committed to prioritizing. It sets up a debate which is currently being argued by the medical profession, by women and by women's organizations, but which individual midwives and the midwifery profession do not seem to be participating in, let alone directing. The debate is about choice; it is about women's freedoms and midwifery autonomy and in order to be fully informed, it needs midwives' voices to be heard. The ten women who are introduced in the next chapter felt that those voices were currently silent.

References

Department of Health and Social Security (1970) Standing Maternity and Midwifery Advisory Committee (J. Peel, Chairman) *Domiciliary Midwifery and Maternity Bed Needs*. London: HMSO.

Department of Health (1993) *Changing Childbirth (Cumberlege Report): Report of the Expert Maternity Group*. London: HMSO.

Department of Health (2007) *Maternity Matters: Choice, access and continuity of care in a safe service*. London: DH.

Lincoln, A. (1863) Gettysburg address, a speech during the American Civil War at the dedication of the soldiers' national cemetery, 19 November.

Luhrmann, B. (1998) *Everybody's free (to wear sunscreen)*. Based on Schmich, M. (1997) Advice, like youth, probably just wasted on the young. Chicago Tribune, 1st June.

Merialdi M. (2010) Women create life. International Conference on Birth and Primal Health, Gran Canaria, 28 February.

National Childbirth Trust (2009) *Location, location, location: Making choice of place of birth a reality*. London: NCT.

Olsen O. and Jewell D. (1998) Home versus hospital birth. *Cochrane Database of Systematic Reviews*, Issue 3.

Tew M. (1986) Do obstetric intranatal interventions make birth safer? *British Journal of Obstetrics and Gynaecology*, 93(7):659–74.

Websites

United Nations Population Fund: Bangladesh: www.unfpa-bangladesh.org/php/thematic_motherhood.php (accessed 31 March 2010).

World Values Survey: www.worldvaluessurvey.org (accessed 17 March 2010).

2 Choosing home birth against medical advice

Much has been written about why women choose home birth (e.g. Pilley Edwards 2005; Viisainen 2001), and this book aims to revisit that topic only briefly in this chapter. The women whose stories are interwoven through the following chapters are unusual because they chose to have their babies at home when doctors and midwives advised them not to. The issues their stories raise are to do with defining normality and risk in childbirth; they highlight uncomfortable issues to do with bullying and coercion in the health service; they demonstrate the serious consequences of iatrogenic stress on maternal well-being and the huge importance of receiving support and encountering empathy when making decisions that are contested by powerful institutions. These stories illustrate the immense complexity of providing care that is truly holistic. None of these issues is uncharted territory; all have figured in the literature. However, these women's stories throw everything into particularly sharp relief, providing raw insights revealing how midwives, doctors and women interact when all parties believe that key principles are at stake.

This chapter introduces the women to you, explaining their childbearing and medical histories, and why they ran into opposition when they declared their intention to have their babies at home. They are all remarkable women, as will become apparent through the following chapters, and they deserve to be known as individuals, rather than merely through disjointed extracts from their stories.

I have not used their real names; this was my agreement with them. The pseudonyms I have chosen for them are popular female names across Europe. I have done this to avoid the inevitable tendency to associate names which are very familiar to us in our own community with certain 'types' or 'classes' of people. As the names are 'foreign', I hope readers will be able to approach the women's stories without being weighed down, even if unconsciously, by the associations which we tend inevitably to make with English names. I also wanted to make the important point that the things that happened to these women matter to all women living in parts of the world where 'Freedom and Choice in Childbirth' (Kitzinger 1988) is not perhaps as transparent as we might wish or believe it to be.

Lea

Lea's first pregnancy resulted from a third cycle of IVF. She wanted a water birth for this very precious baby. Her local hospitals were able to provide a pool, but each hospital had only one. While visiting the hospitals, Lea got the impression that the midwives did not encourage women to use the pools which were, consequently, rarely occupied. Nevertheless, she was anxious about the availability of a pool for her labour, and so started to look into the possibility of hiring one to take into hospital with her. In the course of her enquiries, she came across the local Home Birth Support Group. She and her husband were very moved by the passion of the women they met at the group and although the idea of a home birth had never crossed their minds before, they decided that the most likely way to achieve the normal birth in water that they wanted was to have their baby at home.

Lea had a long-diagnosed heart murmur and her antenatal care was being provided by a consultant who specialized in complex pregnancies. This consultant referred her to a cardiologist when she expressed her desire for a home birth and the cardiologist called a meeting of a team of obstetricians. Everybody present was happy for her to have a home birth.

Towards the end of her pregnancy, Lea began to suffer from itchy feet and palms. Six days before her due date, her waters broke. She asked for expectant management rather than immediate induction of labour. Three days later, she had a positive blood test and there followed what she described as 'very, very hard meetings' with the consultant who insisted she be induced. She resisted and finally went into labour on the day after her due date.

Her labour lasted 24 hours including 8 hours from full dilatation to the birth of her baby boy.

Lili

Lili became pregnant with her first baby on her honeymoon. At her appointment with the midwife, she was told very firmly that she couldn't have a home birth because she lived on an island in the middle of a river and her house was accessible only by foot along a tow path. She repeated her request for a home birth at subsequent appointments until, by 20 weeks, she realized that she was not going to get any support from the local midwives. Her sister who is the mother of four children then suggested to her that she might employ an independent midwife. Lili and her husband decided that this was the right course for them to take, although it was very hard for them to find the money to pay the midwife's fee. When she was two weeks overdue, Lili came under considerable pressure from hospital staff to be induced but she held out and her baby son was born at home in a pool, twenty days after her due date.

Maria-Sofie

Maria-Sofie planned to have her first baby in hospital until, late in her pregnancy, the hospital was stricken with norovirus and, fearing that her husband might be excluded from the postnatal ward and unable to visit her and his new baby, she decided to change her booking to a home birth. She came under pressure to be induced when she was ten days overdue, but remained at home using a birth pool until 'failure to progress', apparently due to dehydration, was diagnosed by her midwife and she was transferred to hospital for the final 45 minutes of her labour.

During her second pregnancy, Maria-Sofie was invited to have a routine HIV tests which she declined. The altercation with her midwife that followed her refusal (an incident described later in this book) led Maria-Sofie to employ an independent midwife and to choose home birth again. At 32 weeks of pregnancy, she was diagnosed with a urine infection and a swab taken by her GP tested positive for group B strep. At this point, she was told by her doctor that she could no longer have a home birth.

With some difficulty, Maria-Sofie persuaded the GP to prescribe antibiotics for the independent midwife to administer to her at home. In the event, the antibiotics were never used because the labour was fast and Maria-Sofie's baby boy was born while the medication was in the process of being drawn up.

Erin

Erin's first pregnancy happened when she was very young and her baby girl was diagnosed *in utero* with a rare condition incompatible with life. Erin and her partner made the heartbreaking decision to have a late termination at 28 weeks. Erin felt that she could not go through an induction and vaginal birth, the course of action preferred by her consultant, and chose instead a general anaesthetic caesarean despite medical concerns about the lack of lower segment development at this stage of pregnancy.

Ten years later and with a new partner, she became pregnant again and miscarried at ten weeks. She had a dilatation and curretage. Her third pregnancy was uneventful, although Erin was naturally very anxious until she had passed the two dates at which she had lost her previous babies. As a result of the sadness she associated with hospital birth, she decided she wanted to have her baby at home, but met with immediate opposition when she first suggested this to her midwife. Erin approached the Supervisor of Midwives and was finally allocated a midwife happy to support her to have a home birth.

Her pregnancy progressed beyond 42 weeks and she came under pressure from the supervisor to agree to an induction. She declined and her 9lbs 4 oz little girl was born at home in water at 43 weeks.

Leonie

Leonie has been living with HIV for ten years and has also suffered from tuberculosis. She has enjoyed excellent health, however, for a long time. She became pregnant when she was 39 years old and was placed under obstetric care. In preparation for her baby, she attended a hypnobirthing course and was strongly influenced by the women whom she met on the course who had chosen to have a home birth.

She and her husband decided that they, too, would like a home birth. Her HIV consultant was fiercely opposed to the idea and was supported in this by Leonie's GP and her obstetrician.

Leonie hired an independent midwife and her baby boy was born at home, 28 hours after her waters had broken.

Mia

Mia's first daughter was born by caesarean after a failed induction for pre-eclampsia. She planned to have her second baby at home, but again developed high blood pressure and reluctantly agreed to have her baby in hospital where she gave birth to her 9lbs 12oz baby boy. Afterwards, she bled heavily and her notes record that she had a postpartum haemorrhage. A year later, she became pregnant again and again asked for a home birth. This was opposed by her consultant, not because of Mia's previous caesarean and haemorrhage, but on the grounds that the baby could be expected to be big. Terrified of hospitals following two very negative experiences, Mia insisted on a home birth. Her labour lasted seven hours and her little boy weighed 10lbs.

Seventeen months later, Mia was pregnant with her fourth child and decided that she would like to have her baby in a birthing pool at home. Her request went to the Supervisor of Midwives who informed her that home water birth was not a service provided in the area. After protracted and unpleasant negotiations, Mia was attended at home by two community midwives who volunteered to care for her. Her labour was slow, and lasted on and off for four days; this was later explained by the fact that her son was born in the direct occipent posterior (OP) position.

Alessia

Alessia's first baby was born in hospital after a straightforward labour lasting four hours. Her second baby was born three years later, this time at home and again without complications. By the time she was pregnant with her third child, however, local consultants' previously favourable attitudes towards home birth had undergone a change and Alessia was told that she should not give birth at home. This advice hardened when Alessia was found to be too large for that date, and investigation revealed only two vessels in the umbilical cord. Nonetheless, she went ahead with the home birth, supported by the local midwives, and her little girl was born safely. While the baby's Apgar scores were excellent and ultrasound scans in the first weeks of her life detected no abnormalities, she was developmentally delayed at two years of age and continues to suffer with problems affecting her balance.

Alessia's fourth pregnancy was unexpected. The baby was again born at home under the care of the same midwives who had supported her in her third labour. At the start of the next pregnancy, a home birth was agreed until the 12 weeks scan revealed twins. Opposition to the home birth from the Supervisor of Midwives was subsequently forceful. As a result of posting on a yahoo group, Alessia and her husband were contacted by two independent midwives who volunteered to support her. A much-reduced fee was agreed because Alessia's husband had just been made redundant and the family was in difficult financial circumstances.

The labour lasted one and a half hours and Alessia gave birth at term to a son weighing 6lbs 8oz and fourteen minutes later, to a daughter weighing 5lbs 7oz.

Margret

Margret's first three babies were born in hospital. All of these labours were induced. Margret is 5'2" tall and her third baby weighed 10lbs 1oz. While Margret's consultant was happy to agree to a home birth for her fourth child, her midwives were very concerned on the grounds that this child was likely to be heavier than the previous one. The pressure from the Supervisor of Midwives for Margret to agree to a hospital delivery was so relentless that she was driven to contemplate free birthing. Finally, she was able to get the support of an independent midwife. This midwife wanted another colleague to assist her, and a friend of Margret's agreed to be the second midwife. Margret's baby boy was born at 40 weeks + 5 days and weighed 9lbs exactly.

Mette

Mette's first baby was born at home. She sustained a third degree tear and lost a lot of blood. Her recovery from this injury was very slow and Mette had to work hard with the help of a physiotherapist to regain the normal functioning of her pelvic floor. Just over a year later, she became pregnant again and was offered a caesarean section on the grounds that this would protect her anal sphincter as a vaginal birth might result in another serious tear. She decided against elective surgery, and with the support of a local midwife, chose once again to have a home birth. The Supervisor of Midwives opposed her decision, citing increased risk of postpartum haemorrhage. Mette insisted and a birth plan was put in place, stating that the labour must be attended by a senior midwife. When Mette was in strong labour, her partner rang for a midwife but Mette's daughter was born while a senior midwife was still being sought to attend the birth.

Romaně

Romaně's first baby was born in hospital after 48 hours of labour. Being on the delivery suite did not enable Romaně and her partner to have the intimate private experience that they felt was very important for them while bringing a child into the world. During her next pregnancy, Romaně made the decision to have no health professionals with her in labour. She spent the first stage in water and moved to her bedroom to give birth to her daughter following a four hours labour.

Why did the women choose home birth?

Although this book is not primarily about what motivated the women to choose home birth, but rather about what happened to them when they did make this choice, their reasons naturally form an important part of their stories. Yet there is no simple answer to the question of why they made their decision and stuck to it in the face of heavy opposition. The influences which operate on our decisions, whether they are relatively unimportant decisions or life-changing, are complex and defy any attempt to reduce them to discrete categories. The essence of holistic care is to appreciate that any woman's approach to birth is coloured by a complex interplay of factors. Prominent among these are likely to be her previous life experiences, her personality, her attitude towards risk (which will be influenced by a combination of the two previous factors), her relationship with her own body – how she feels about it, whether she likes it, whether she trusts it – and the extent to which she accepts authority outside herself. This may well depend on her upbringing, on the kind of schooling she has had, and on whether she has found authority figures to be trustworthy and attractive or untrustworthy and unattractive. When she becomes pregnant, whether for the first or the tenth time, she is never an 'obstetric object' but 'a person with hopes and fears, views and opinions, personality and relationships, within a unique social context' (Methven 1989). She is a Hamlet figure, as we all are; someone who is ultimately unknowable. To presume to know her better than she knows herself is to demean her:

> Why, look you now, how unworthy a thing you make of me! You would play upon me; you would seem to know my stops; you would pluck out the heart of my mystery; you would sound me from my lowest note to the top of my compass . . . do you think I am easier to be played on than a pipe?
>
> (Shakespeare, *Hamlet*, Act 3, Scene 2:356–360; 362–363)

No single factor explains the choice made by any of the women whose stories are outlined above. However, to tease out some of the influences which acted upon them may enable the decisions made by other women to be better understood, women with similarly complicated medical histories which common sense suggests would propel them into hospital at the very first twinge of labour.

First and foremost, all of these women wanted a *natural* birth. It may be that this is less and less important to women today, although I am inclined to think that many would love to enjoy the sense of achievement that doing it 'all on their own' would create. For the women in this book, the link between the way in which they gave birth, and their self-esteem and self-concept, was particularly strong. Even if it was their first baby, they knew that the birth they had was going to affect the kind of woman they were, for the rest of their lives. This is what Penny Simkin (1991; 1992) found in her famous research which explored older women's recollections of their childbirth experiences. Simkin discovered that women's memories of their first births, even as long as 40 years later, were accurate, vivid and deeply felt. Women who recalled their births with satisfaction described an ongoing sense of achievement which had constantly bolstered their self-esteem and confidence during their lives. The women in this book felt very strongly that they could not achieve in hospital an experience which would impact positively on their emotional and spiritual well-being.

They felt that good birth experiences lead to a more fulfilling and straightforward transition into motherhood, so by choosing home birth they were trying to maximize the quality of the relationship they achieved with their baby:

> It struck me that people who had had good birth experiences got on better. People who had bad ones and who had had a lot of interventions seemed to have more problems bonding with their baby and dealing with motherhood.
>
> Lili

Some of the women were very strongly affected by their previous birth experiences and some had reached crisis point in terms of their ability to tolerate even being inside a hospital:

> I couldn't go back to the hospital where my first baby had been born. I found it hard even to drive past it. So we went to look at another birthing unit. And the midwife said, 'I'll show you where the theatre is, just in case'. We went through some double doors and we were walking along, chatting, and I froze and broke down. The smell of going near the theatre was too much. I said, 'I can't do this'.
>
> Mia

Mette had received two units of blood following a traumatic tear during her first birth. In her next pregnancy, she was asked to give a routine blood sample:

> It was the first time that I'd had anything done like that since the blood transfusion. I really couldn't do it, initially, on the spot, even though my husband was with me. The midwives thought I was time wasting and just being stupid because I couldn't do it without mental preparation. I went back at four months and they said, 'We've got to do your blood today' and I thought I had prepared myself for it, but as she started taking my blood, it was a nightmare.
>
> Mette

They chose home birth because it was very important for them to be in control, especially if injury had occurred during a previous labour and they felt this had been due to health professionals trying to control their bodies without fully understanding what the women themselves knew was happening to them:

> I wanted to be in control; I wanted to be able to relax [to avoid another serious tear].
>
> Mette

The depth of women's need to have an experience that would redeem themselves in their own eyes following a difficult previous birth was often apparent:

> I knew other people who had had a similarly traumatic first delivery who had had a fantastic second delivery, and it was a really redeeming experience. I wanted to have a fantastic experience.
>
> Mette

All of the women *knew* – intellectually, physically, psychologically and spiritually – that the decision to have a home birth was the right one for them, and several claimed sisterhood with birthing women down the ages:

> I kept coming back to the same idea and the same belief that this was right for me. Millions of women in the past, for thousand of years, have done this. We are here and this means that our mothers, our grandmothers, our great grandmothers have managed to give birth without the intervention of hospitals.
>
> Alessia

> I've never been so comfortable in a decision I've made.
>
> Lili

They were far too intelligent to subscribe to what has been described as 'the obstetric ideal', which holds out the promise of 'perfect babies' if only women will submit to medical management of their pregnancies and births. They did not accept the 'biomedical hegemony' (Davis-Floyd 1997), which is central to our cultural understanding of childbirth and its presumption that women's bodies are incompetent to birth their babies and require the assistance of professionals to ensure a safe outcome:

> Women are so used to being told that the way their bodies are working is wrong. How can they then trust their instincts?
>
> > Margret

Ironically, these women who chose to have home births *against medical advice* justified their decision using the rhetoric that the government has been proclaiming for years, namely that women should be at the centre of maternity service provision (DH 2007: 7) and that they should be free to make the decisions that are right for them. Following very careful reflection, they came to the conclusion that if they were to be truly powerful in their own labours and births, they must choose the environment which ensured that decision-making would not rest with health professional staff, but would be relocated with them:

> I did consider the hospital, but I knew that if I really wanted to be in a place of power and decision-making, the only place I could do that would be at home.
>
> > Mette

The environment the women wanted for their labours was in keeping with the environment which the radical and highly influential midwife, Tricia Anderson (2002) famously described in a lecture on how cats birth, and the conditions which promote effective labour in mammals:

> Everyone knows that cats need to give birth undisturbed in a dark, secluded place – perhaps preparing a softly lined box in the darkest corner of the furthest room underneath the bed. And everyone who knows about cats understands that you must never disturb a cat in labour or a newly delivered cat and her litter of kittens. Otherwise the cat's labour will stop or she may reject her kittens. Everyone knows this.

> I waddled around the house. We had music on. We lit the candles. It was really dark and quiet and calm.
>
> > Erin

The *safety* that the women felt in their own homes depended on their intuitive conviction that labour would progress normally, and that their babies would be born safely:

I was starting to go into second stage and active pushing. There was some meconium. One of the midwives went straight out to phone for an ambulance. I said, 'I know this baby is OK' and he was born quite soon after that. I knew, I absolutely knew and trusted that this baby was OK.

Mia

They knew that they would be able to cope using their own resources and that their relationship with both their partner and their new baby would be enhanced by being in their own environment. They valued emotional safety (Hunter and Deery 2009) and felt that it was intricately bound up with the physical safety of birth. They argued that physical safety is not necessarily protected by virtue of being in a medical environment. A father (see chapter 7) whose experience of being present at the birth of his son at home changed him from being a home-birth-averse GP to a home birth activist, acknowledged that the compound presentation of his baby would have resulted in a very different kind of birth in hospital from the one which took place at his house:

Lola was between my legs. I have no idea how long we were in that position. Time stretched to infinity yet, at the same time, it was seconds. The midwife said something and I knew it was not a good thing for her to be saying, but by the time I had processed 'compound presentation', I could hear the baby crying and, of course, I burst into tears too ... Had we been in hospital, the moment anyone had detected that the baby had his hand up – buzzers would have been pressed, the room would have been swimming with people – panic – the tachycardia would have prompted the doctor to be called, blood cultures to be ordered. The delayed third stage would have been a manual delivery in theatre – it would have been the most horrible experience.

Jon

The women leaned toward individual, 'subjective and holistic knowledge', as opposed to medical knowledge which does not take into account 'the importance of biological, social, spiritual, cultural and psychological factors' (Hewitt-Taylor 2004: 34). Yet all of them had extensively researched the risks they were perceived by health professionals to be running and had made their choice to birth at home based on understanding the facts as well as on intuition. As Andrews (2004) commented in a recent study of home birth, 'In terms of balancing safety and risk against place of birth, the participants were probably better informed than most women' (p. 521). Some of the women openly challenged the partiality of the evidence on which professionals were basing their assessment of risk:

Alessia: I don't want a caesarean and I don't want to come into hospital.
HP: Do you know that the second twin is five more times likely to die in hospital than a singleton baby?

Alessia: Is that in hospital?

HP: Yes.

Alessia: How on earth is that meant to reassure me then? What's the statistic for home birth?

HP: We haven't got one.

It is not clear why these women were able to resist the 'coercive pull of medicalisation' (Machin and Scamell, cited in Hunter and Deery 2009) and the hegemony of a medical model of birth so powerful that for most women there no longer exists a choice – in so far as that word implies a debate with either oneself or one's carers – about where they should have their babies. It is clear that they wholeheartedly rejected the abrogation of autonomy that contemporary hospital birth renders inevitable. Their frame of mind is summed up by P. D. James in her novel, *The Private Patient* (2008):

> To become a patient was to relinquish a part of oneself, to be received into a system which, however benign, subtly robbed one of initiative, almost of will.
>
> (p. 13)

They were unusual in their refusal to accept that whatever is, is for the best, as described by Porter and Macintyre (1984):

> Pregnant women appeared to assume that whatever arrangements they had experienced were the best arrangements possible and to be negative about innovations until they had experienced them.
>
> (p. 1197)

Houghton and Lavender (2008) note women's 'apathy' (p. 5), their unwilling-ness to challenge professionals and their lack of insight into the possibility that interventions in childbirth might create their own problems even while attempting to solve others. In an earlier study, Kirkham *et al.* (2002) identified women's reluctance to question (p. 509) and their collusion with midwives 'in accepting and maintaining an inequitable and inadequate maternity service' (p. 513). Challenge is the lifeblood of improvement; the challenge that led to the exposure of serious deficiencies in the management of Mid Staffordshire Hospital Trust (www.cqc.org.uk) came, not from within, but from relatives of patients who questioned the practice they were observing on the wards. Questioning is often considered by health professionals to be an indication either of arrogance or of ingratitude on the part of the questioner. It is not necessarily either; it may simply be a means of taking responsibility alongside health professionals for one's own or one's relatives' safety.

Mistakes are frequent in hospitals. In 2008–9, there were 6080 claims against the NHS for clinical negligence; this figure had increased from 5470 claims in the years 2007–8 (National Health Service Litigation Authority). The maternity service cares predominantly for well women and focuses on a normal bodily function, namely giving birth. Any intervention therefore requires robust justification. After all, it is hard to believe that modern obstetrics, which has existed for less than a hundred years, should have got birth more right than evolution, which has been working on it for millennia (Jesus Sanz, Mid-Atlantic Conference 2010). If an assumption were made (theoretically) that one mistake occurs per every 1000 intrapartum interventions, and if each of the 690,000 women who gives birth in the UK each year receives just one intervention, this will result in 690 mistakes of which a proportion will be serious or fatal. If, however, only 1000 interventions are carried out, this would lead to just one mistake, possibly serious, possibly fatal, but probably not. The case for ensuring that every intervention is therefore totally justified seems irrefutable.

The strength of a democratic institution lies in its ability to recognize and celebrate diversity of opinion; it is tolerance of difference that contributes to the happiness of a nation (World Values Survey). Monolithic institutions, whether financial, legal or health, require constant challenge to ensure that they remain accountable and focussed on the people they were set up to serve. In 2003, Wilmot (cited in Hewitt-Taylor 2004) declared that the age of deference to doctors was coming to an end and that the biomedical model of health was being challenged. If this is the case, it is not immediately apparent in maternity care. A less hopeful viewpoint is captured by Sara Wickham (2007), who comments that while the rights of women to make informed choices about their care is theoretically the corner-stone of the maternity service, 'this would come as a surprise (or even a joke) to most pregnant women' (p. 5). Lynn Walcott, a young midwife, writes online in 2010 about her reasons for leaving the profession she has worked in for only a few years, namely that 'the NHS has seeped into independence' (www.midwifery.org.uk).

There is a strong tendency to label people who refuse to conform to normative practices, such as giving birth in hospital, and to the dominant knowledge system, such as the biomedical model of childbirth, as deviant (Stewart 2001). Those who make mainstream choices feel justified and more confident if other people make the same choices. This is why prophets who challenge the system are never welcome in their own land (Luke 4:24); they are uncomfortable people to live with. Sometimes, however, they get it right.

At the start of the twentieth century, women in Great Britain did not have the vote. The Suffragettes campaigned for this right, using a variety of tactics, some of which drew the censure not only of conservative men but also of their own sex. Today historians argue whether the Suffragettes advanced the cause of female emancipation or delayed it. There seems little doubt, however, that Emmeline Pankhurst and her followers put votes for women on the national agenda. In a political and cultural climate in which Viscount Helmsley could make the following speech in the House of Commons, one can but feel that women had to act:

> The way in which certain types of women, easily recognised, have acted in the last year or two . . . lends a great deal of colour to the argument

that the mental equilibrium of the female sex is not as stable as the mental equilibrium of the male sex . . . one feels that it is not cricket for women to use force . . . it is little short of nauseating and disgusting to the whole sex.

(28 March 1912)

The women whose stories are told in this book met with open hostility and some ridicule from friends and professionals when they chose to have their babies at home. The rate of home birth in the UK remains low, at 2.7 per cent in 2008 (www.birthchoiceuk.com); if choice of place of birth was more openly and wholeheartedly offered, it is thought that 16 per cent of women would consider giving birth at home (MORI poll commissioned by the Expert Maternity Group, DH 1993). It is not clear whether these 16 per cent would be the women who 'ought' to choose it. The 16 per cent might perhaps include women who would choose home birth despite being considered unsuitable candidates owing to their previous obstetric histories or current medical condition. Is this a problem? The following chapters explore how a highly controlling health service invested strongly in defending itself against dissenters. Whether one thinks that the women were misguided or enlightened in the decisions that they took, they have unwittingly benefitted the maternity service by challenging it to justify the premises on which it operates.

Key points

- The strength of a democratic institution lies in its ability to recognize and celebrate diversity of opinion.
- Holistic care depends on appreciating that a woman's approach to birth is individual and coloured by a complex interplay of factors.
- It is reasonable to assume that a good birth experience may lead to a more fulfilling and straightforward transition to motherhood.
- Women who refuse to accept that whatever is, is for the best, are those who can transform the maternity service.

References

Anderson T. (2002) Out of the laboratory: back to the darkened room. *MIDIRS Midwifery Digest*, 21(1):65–69.

Andrews A. (2004) Home birth experience 1: decision and expectation. *British Journal of Midwifery*, 12(8):518–523.

Davis-Floyd (1997) *Childbirth and Authoritative Knowledge*. Berkeley: University of California Press.

Department of Health (1993) *Changing Childbirth (Cumberlege Report): Report of the Expert Maternity Group*. London: HMSO.

Department of Health (2007) *Maternity Matters: Choice, access and continuity of care in a safe service*. London: HMSO.

Helmsley Viscount C. W. (1912) Debate on the 'Conciliation Bill'. Official Reports 5th Series Parliamentary Debates: Commons, Vol xxxvi (Mar 25–Apr 12, 1912) cols 615–732.

Hewitt-Taylor J. (2004) Challenging the balance of power: patient empowerment. *Nursing Standard*, 18(22):33–37.

Houghton G. and Lavender T. (2008) Factors influencing choice in birth place: an exploration of the views of women, their partners and professionals. *Evidence Based Midwifery*, June, available online at www.rcm.org.uk (accessed 17 March 2010).

Hunter B. and Deery R. (2009) *Emotions in Midwifery and Reproduction*. Basingstoke: Palgrave Macmillan.

James P. D. (2008) *The Private Patient*. London: Penguin Books.

Kirkham M., Stapleton H., Curtis P. and Thomas G. (2002) The inverse care law in antenatal midwifery care. *British Journal of Midwifery*, 10(8):509–513.

Kitzinger S. (1988) *Freedom and Choice in Childbirth*. London: Penguin Books.

Methven R. (1989) Recording an obstetric history or relating to a pregnant woman? A study of the antenatal booking interview. In: Robinson S. and Thomson A. M. (eds) *Midwives, Research and Childbirth 1*. London: Chapman and Hall: 42–71.

Pilley Edwards N. (2005) *Birthing Autonomy: Women's experiences of planning home births*. London: Routledge.

Porter M. and Macintyre S. (1984) What is, must be best: a research note on conservative or deferential responses to antenatal care provision. *Social Science and Medicine*, 19(11):1197–1200.

Sanz J. (2010) Roundtable Discussion, *Childbirth in 2050*. International Conference on Birth and Primal Health, Gran Canaria, 28 February, 2010.

Shakespeare W. (1969) *Hamlet* (Edited by Rylands G.) Oxford: Clarendon Press (New Clarendon Shakespeare).

Simkin P. (1991) Just another day in a woman's life? Women's long-term perceptions of their first birth experience. *Birth*, 18(4):203–210.

Simkin P. (1992) Just another day in a woman's life? Women's long-term perceptions of their first birth experience. *Birth*, 19(2):64–81.

Stewart M. (2001) Whose evidence counts? An exploration of health professionals' perceptions of evidence-based practice, focusing on the maternity services. *Midwifery*, 17:280.

Viisainen K. (2001) Negotiating control and meaning: home birth as a self-constructed choice in Finland. *Social Science and Medicine*, 52:1109–1121.

Wickham S. (2007) *'What's right for me?' Making decisions in pregnancy and birth* (2nd ed.) Association for Improvements in the Maternity Services.

Websites

BirthChoiceUK: www.birthchoiceuk.com/BirthChoiceUKFrame.htm? www.birthchoice uk.com/HomeBirthRates.htm (accessed 18 April 2010).

Lynn Walcott: www.midwifery.org.uk/123lynnwalcott.htm (accessed 10 March 2010).

Mid-Staffordshire NHS Foundation Trust: www.cqc.org.uk/usingcareservices/health care/concernsabouthealthcare/midstaffordshirenhsfoundationtrust.cfm (accessed 14 March 2010).

National Health Service Litigation Authority: www.nhsla.com/home.htm (accessed 16 March 2010).

World Values Survey: www.worldvaluessurvey.org (accessed 17 March 2010).

3 Fear and risk

Antenatal classes are a good opportunity to gauge expectant parents' attitudes and beliefs about labour and birth. Over the 25 years that I have been working in education for parenthood, I have noticed a steady escalation in the fear that women feel about birthing their babies. It is hard to know whether their fear has grown in line with the increase in screening and surveillance to which pregnancy is now subjected, or whether it is their fear that has generated the increased medical surveillance. Either way, pregnant women's sense of self-efficacy, of being able to take charge of their lives, and control events in relation to birth, appears to have diminished significantly.

In the introduction to this book, it was suggested that the happiness of nations might depend on people's perception of having a variety of choices in their lives and being free to choose among them (World Values Survey). When asked how they would like to give birth to their babies, expectant mothers will very often respond, 'I'd love to do it all myself, without any drugs, *if I could*', and the response to a question about their preferred method of feeding their babies is, 'I'd like to breastfeed, *if I can*'. On the one hand is their statement about the choice they would like to make, and on the other, the statement that immediately nullifies that choice, the 'get-out' clause that gives permission either not to make the choice at all or not to achieve it if they do make it.

The overwhelming atmosphere in antenatal classes today is one of fear – fear of two kinds. Firstly, there is fear of making choices, because the choices people most want are the choices they feel are least likely to be realized; this is the ancient sense of *hubris*, tempting fate by presuming to aim for something that is beyond your reach, a presumption that in mythological terms brings down the wrath of the gods. The second fear is of labour and birth itself, a fear of what are perceived to be the huge risks involved and an accompanying sense of the need to be rescued from nature by technology and medical expertise.

It is tempting, and perhaps not unreasonable, to speculate that the increase in tokophobia or pathological fear of childbirth is related, at least in part, to its removal from the domestic arena to the medical, from home to hospital, and from the control of women to the control of doctors. Ten years ago, the Daily Mail (Koster 2001) quoted Dr Kristina Hofberg as saying that some women's 'intense dread and avoidance of childbirth' could lead them to take such extreme action as 'abusing alcohol or drugs, or punching their own abdomen in an effort to abort the child'. Interestingly, such women were also reported as having 'a lack of trust in their obstetric team' which begs the question of why they considered 'an obstetric team' to be an inevitable part of childbirth.

The tension that characterizes contemporary antenatal education is the tension between parents' 'choice talk' which goes on at the cognitive level and a far deeper, emotional discourse where they unwittingly betray that choices around childbirth are not real to them. This can be seen, for example, in the lack of congruence between their intellectual understanding of what constitutes a good birth environment and their emotional rejection of the suggestion that home might be that perfect birth environment. Ask both women and men to draw their ideal birth place and they will produce a picture in which soft surfaces abound – easy chairs, deep pile rugs, mountains of cushions, low large beds piled with pillows – where the lighting is low, where there is an absence of people and an abundance of food and drink. Ask them next whether home might be the most likely place to find or create such an environment and they will nod sadly, and move on to enquiring how many pillows there are in the delivery rooms at the local hospital. The environment their instincts crave is one described by Mia:

> We had the birth pool in the front room. We sealed the front door which leads into this room. Nobody was coming in or going out of the house from there because I needed a safe, enclosed room. We took the TV and anything like that out, and we just had a birth pool and some chairs. Once I was in the pool, everybody went out. I felt I would be best by myself. I didn't want to be watched by people. The whole labour was very quiet.

Hospital is perceived as a place of safety because labour and birth are perceived to be so risky and risk is perceived to be minimized through medical intervention. Ask a group of men attending antenatal classes whether women are able to give birth unaided, and they will be very doubtful. It is generally pointless for the childbirth educator, either in the interests of helping people to have a better, more humane birth, or simply in the interests of accuracy, to give the evidence that increasing intervention rates have not made labour and birth any safer, that as the caesarean section rates have risen and risen, neonatal mortality rates have not improved. Figures for mortality rates tend to appear several years after the period to which they refer. The diagram below describes trends for 1995 to 2003 and is related to the figures published for the same period by the Confidential Enquiry into Maternal and Child Health (RCOG 2005).

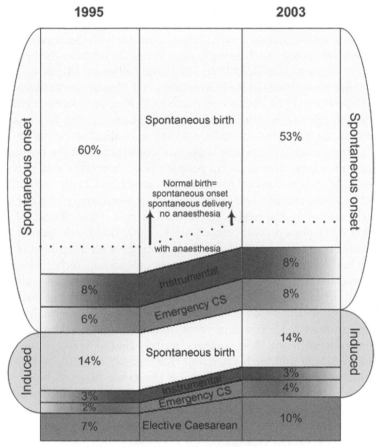

Figure 3.1   Trends in Childbirth.
Source: BirthChoiceUK: www.birthchoiceuk.com/Professionals/index.html

Confidential Enquiry into Maternal and Child Health (2005) *Stillbirth, Neonatal and Post-neonatal Mortality 2000–3, England, Wales and Northern Ireland.* London: RCOG Press.

Key findings

- A significant increase in the stillbirth rate in England, Wales and Northern Ireland was seen from 2001 to 2002. This increase was sustained in 2003.
- A small increase in the neonatal mortality rate was seen from 2002 to 2003.

At a recent international conference on childbirth, a representative of the World Health Organization demonstrated to a still sceptical audience of mid-wives and obstetricians that a caesarean section rate of above 15 per cent has no impact on maternal mortality and that countries with the heaviest reliance on obstetric technology, such as the United States, do not have the best neona-tal mortality figures (Merialdi 2010). The Royal College of Midwives' position paper *Home Birth* (2002) quotes Campbell's and Macfarlane's seminal work, *Where to be Born* (1994), observing that 'the iatrogenic risks associated with institutional delivery, which are often overlooked . . . may be equal to or greater than the benefit of immediate access to medical attention' (p. 1).

Just as the choices that people make are constructed on the basis of infi-nitely complex motivations, so are people's fears. It is often said that health professionals' perceptions of the risks of labour and birth are fuelled by fear of litigation, and this fear is justified in an increasingly litigious society where claims for clinical negligence in the UK rose in the period 2008/9 to £769,000,000 from a previous record of £633,000,000 for the period 2007/8 (www.nhsla.com). Stapleton *et al.* (2002) note the widespread belief among obstetric health professionals that in the event of litigation, technological inter-vention in childbirth (rather than no intervention) will be viewed positively by judges and juries. The authors consider that this reinforces notions of there being 'right' and 'wrong' choices rather than 'informed' choices (p. 639).

Health professional fear is dependent on the same cultural beliefs as those that control women and their partners, namely that technology and surveil-lance make labour and birth safer, and that as hospital is the natural home of medical technology, hospital must be the safest place to birth. This is an entirely reasonable position to hold when personal experience has been principally, if not exclusively, of labour complications occurring in hospital. The words of one of the fathers, a GP, interviewed for this book summarize a common professional viewpoint:

> I'd always envisaged home birth as being slightly hippy, a slightly crazy thing for women to do and if patients requested a home birth, I'd say, 'Well, if that's what you want to do, then so be it, but I really wouldn't rec-ommend it'. And I said that on the basis of anecdote and having worked in a large teaching obstetric centre and seeing endless complications.
>
> Leon

> Most professionals agreed their professional experience, dealing with emergencies and complications, had increased their perception of risk. This negatively affected their views of birth away from the hospital facilities.
>
> (Houghton and Lavender 2008)

Health professionals may be as vulnerable to an aberrant childbirth mythology which they create from the stories they tell each other, as are women. The public taste for television which depicts medical dramas indicates that there is a profound need to add colour to our generally very safe lives by watching life and death situations, people experiencing extreme emotions and doctors demonstrating superb skills to rescue patients from horrendous injuries, very rare diseases and, in the case of childbirth, multiple births and shoulder dystocia. The most frequently viewed television programme globally in 2008 was *House*, a medical drama starring Hugh Laurie as a brilliant diagnostician whose hospital allows him a team of three doctors to handle just one 'medical mystery' per working week. Each episode concludes with a patient being diagnosed with a condition so rare or so unlikely in his or her age and social group that 99 per cent of doctors will never experience the like over a lifetime of practice.

If I go to postnatal groups where women meet to tell their birth stories, the stories are charged with emotion, but often the emotions described are not those which occurred when the women brought their babies into the world, but are the emotions associated with a fraught journey to hospital once labour was underway, the consultations with midwives and doctors about 'what to do', and as likely as not, the dash to theatre for an assisted delivery or caesarean section. Knowledge of childbirth is thus constructed through social interaction among women just as human interaction is the basis of creating and legitimizing all knowledge, according to Vygotsky (1978). By telling the particular kinds of stories they do, women unwittingly 'teach' other women that childbirth is dangerous and 'fearful' – literally, 'full of fear'. Midwives tell each other the same kind of stories couched in professional terms and so the mythology of risk and rescue is created and sustained.

Risk management is, therefore, as Denis Walsh (2003) notes, never 'objective'. Rather it is 'socially constructed, biased to certain values and politically motivated to reinforce the powerful in health care' (p. 474). The power-base in maternity care remains in hospitals, unlike for example, in mental health services where the power-base now lies in the community. This leads to a distorted perception of who or what is to blame should problems arise. If a baby dies in hospital, it is assumed that everything possible was done by health professionals to prevent that tragedy from occurring, and that the tragedy was therefore inevitable; on the other hand, if a baby dies at home, it is immediately presumed that negligence and/or irresponsibility on the part of the midwife or mother must be a significant factor (Beech 2009). Health professionals consider (probably correctly) that most newspapers read by 'ordinary people' and most disciplinary panels, will assess quality of care according to level of technological intervention, and that the right professional choice (with consequent limitations on the women's choices) is to use the technology (Stapleton *et al.* 2002).

It is common that if a country feels itself to be under threat, people's choices may be constrained until the threat is perceived to have passed (increasingly invasive and intrusive airport security in the UK and USA is one example of an intrusive response to the perceived threat of terrorism, but one which most people would consider necessary). Similarly, in a health care system which is obsessed with the prevention of litigation rather than on the promotion of well-being, the autonomy of the individual (whether clinician or client) may be limited or abolished (Furedi 2006). In the maternity services, the climate of insecurity means that there is a gulf between the rhetoric of choice on the one hand, and the reality of risk management on the other, or to put it another way, there is a vigorous (and unresolved) debate between professional duty of care and women's choice (Kingdon *et al.* 2003).

There have long been Risk Management Midwives in post; the title of the post betrays the attitude towards pregnancy and birth: birth is risky – to women, to midwives' careers and to hospital budgets. At a recent study-day run by CMACE (Centre for Maternal and Child Enquiries), a midwife running an antenatal clinic spoke of how the risk-assessment tool used in her hospital was now so refined that it was difficult for any woman to achieve a low-risk label. She presented this information as an indicator of the quality of care provided to pregnant women in her area, a remarkable indicator of the distance obstetrics has travelled in the half century since the American surgeon, Montgomery, speaking on the normality of birth in 1958, pronounced:

> I have stated on numerous occasions that there is no more need to interfere with the course of normally progressing labour than there is to tamper with good digestion, normal respiration and adequate circulation.

Very accurate risk-assessment tools are, however, notoriously inaccurate. Common sense tells us that women whose pregnancies are labelled as 'high-risk' often have straightforward and uneventful labours and births, and women labelled as 'low-risk' run into difficulties. Commenting on various scoring tools used in maternity services in the USA, Jordan and Murphy (2009) describe their validity as 'undetermined', and conclude:

> When women are placed in risk categories based on tools with poor predictive value for actual occurrence of complications, this categorization can mislead care decisions. A recent analysis of 12 scoring tools to predict pre-term birth found the tool performed poorly and resulted in more frequent hospitalizations and interventions in the group labelled 'at-risk' with no significant improvement in pre-term birth rates.
>
> (p. 192)

In their joint statement on home birth, the Royal College of Midwives and the Royal College of Obstetricians and Gynaecologists (2007) acknowledge that there are no risk-assessment tools that are effective in predicting the outcomes of labour.

Pushed to the extreme, risk management becomes an absurdity. This is recognized by ordinary people in their everyday conversation when they comment wryly on instances of 'health and safety gone mad' in relation to the latest edict from government, local authorities, the workplace, schools or the Department of Health about what they should or should not be allowed to do in order to be kept safe. A less obsessive focus on risk is welcomed by many British tourists when they travel to countries in Europe or farther afield where people are free to behave in ways that would cause them to fall foul of the law in the UK (such as placing ladders against trees and carrying children on the handle bars of their bicycles). In a speech given at a midwifery conference in Manchester in 2005 which drew prolonged applause from an audience of midwives who recognized all too clearly the kind of farce which the speaker was describing, Ruth Sharples Weston (2005) reported the words of the midwife sent to support her during a home water birth that had been fiercely resisted by her consultant:

[Ruth's labour moves into second stage; the midwife steps forward.]

'At this moment, I have to ask you to leave the pool as it is not the Trust's policy to allow you to remain in the pool for the birth'. I politely refused and proceeded to give birth in the pool unimpeded – but what a farce! So even though my consultant was not present at my NHS birth, he was present in the actions and words of the midwives who were.

The stage at which risk assessment tips into absurdity is illustrated by Margret's account of an incident in her home birth saga:

[The Supervisor of Midwives visits Margret to give her a document to be included in her hand-held notes.]

This stated that I had to have an ambulance outside as soon as I was in labour; I had to have a venflon sited in second stage; not only did I have to have two community midwives with me during labour, but a Supervisor of Midwives was to be called and present for 'documentation purposes'. The hospital closest to me had to be notified that I was in labour, and also the other hospital which I am quite close to so that in an emergency, the ambulance people could choose which one to take me to. The Head of Midwifery at both units had to be informed that I was in labour.

The mother's reaction was not unsurprising:

I thought, 'Oh my goodness, this is over the top', and I spent the rest of the day crying.

Margret

Another mother exposed the inconsistency between different units' approaches to managing risk:

They told me on day 9 that I would have to be induced on day 10. I asked for the medical reason and they said that it was their policy.

I saw three different consultants who tried to get me to be induced. And none of them could give me a reason other than that it was their policy. So then I asked, 'Well, if your policy is 10 days, why is the policy at W. hospital, down the road, 14 days? They couldn't answer; they just said it was – policy.

Maria-Sofie

Margret was designated 'at risk' because she had previously given birth to three large babies and it was assumed that the fourth would be even larger. Perceptions of this risk varied from health professional to health professional:

a)   The consultant was very open. She didn't try to scare me at all. She said, 'there's a very small risk that you will have shoulder dystocia. It could happen in hospital as much as at home, but in hospital we have paediatricians'. However, she wrote on my notes that she had no objection to my having a home birth.

b)   I continued to 38 weeks with the midwives every now and again hinting that this baby was huge and it was going to be 11 lbs.

c)   I have a friend who's a midwife and I asked her to have a feel of my tummy and she said, 'It feels like a good size baby, Margret, but it doesn't feel huge'.

While distressed by these conflicting viewpoints, Margret decided that her own knowledge was likely to be the most accurate:

I *knew* I wasn't as big as I had been with my last.

Erin got to 42 weeks in her pregnancy, and was well aware that there are slight risks with prolonged pregnancy. A variety of factors caused her to assess her risk as being low, so that she was able to resist the scaremongering of professional staff:

a)   The twice weekly EFM monitoring and the scans showed that everything was normal; the baby was fine and I was fine; the placenta wasn't giving up and everything was great.

b)   I was pretty sure I wasn't overdue anyway because I have long menstrual cycles, sometimes between 33 and 36 days.

c)   My mum told me I was born at about 42 weeks myself and I felt like this might have some bearing on my pregnancy. So I wasn't worried.

The midwives' risk assessment, quite reasonably, was based on what they were familiar with from their own practice which was limited by Trust policy. Their knowledge of prolonged pregnancy was circumscribed because the women they cared for were routinely induced at 40 weeks + 10 days:

By 42 weeks, the community midwives were saying that they had never met a lady who'd gone further than 42 weeks. They were in effect saying that I was pretty much a freak of nature as far as their practice was concerned.

Erin

The women in this book did not ignore the risks they were told they were running; quite the reverse. They researched them in depth, and then reached their own conclusions:

I started looking on the internet every day. I researched breech birth and twin birth and the complications. I created a huge folder for myself. I looked at Mary Cronk and Jane Evans. I was on the UK Midwifery Forum. I would email different midwives quite regularly, asking them questions, asking them about their experiences. As time went on, I was thinking, 'I still believe this is right for me'.

Alessia

Mette's goal with her second baby was to avoid another serious tear such as had occurred with her first baby, and from which she had suffered prolonged pain and psychological distress. In order to minimize her risk, she decided:

It came down to being able to relax; that seemed to me the most important thing, to avoid tensing up. For me to relax, I needed to be somewhere like my own house.

Her risk assessment was that being at home was likely to be more effective as a strategy for avoiding a third degree tear than being in hospital.

In addition to carrying out their own assessments of their individual circumstances, the women were also aware of risks that affect every woman's labour and these formed part of their decision-making:

I knew lots of reasons why things go wrong when women go into hospital. When adrenaline kicks in, it stops the production of oxytocin; when you get scared, things go wrong and then interventions happen.

Alessia

The credibility and authority accorded to risk management rests on its appeal to the 'evidence-base'. The health service insists that its clinicians' work must be directed and rendered accountable by its adherence to evidence. Interestingly, so powerful in the public consciousness is the idea of 'evidence' that even voluntary organizations which have traditionally based their credibility on the appeal to *experiential* knowledge, have incorporated the 'evidence-base' into their manifestos and public statements:

We have a range of policy briefings and position statements which set out what we believe, together with the relevant research evidence.

The NCT contributes to the development of national policies working with government departments for the UK, England, Northern Ireland, Scotland and Wales. We help to develop evidence-based guidelines, in collaboration with professional bodies and the National Institute for Health & Clinical Excellence (NICE).

(National Childbirth Trust 2010)

However, for every research study that finds itself in favour of one treatment, there is, of course, another that finds no advantage in its use. The evidence is always in a state of *becoming*; it is a chrysalis turning into a butterfly, but never a fully fledged butterfly. The same evidence can give rise to passionate debate from opposing disinterested experts and from opposing interested parties. There is no harm in this; indeed, it is the debate and the ongoing questioning that strengthens or develops the evidence. The human animal is an enquiring one; every research paper ends with suggestions for further research on the basis that the evidence presented in the paper is inevitably partial. Recent media coverage of various health-related scandals has well and truly demonstrated that the evidence-base is as subject to human imperfection as anything else. As this book was being written, the newspapers were full of the scandal surrounding Avandia, the drug used to treat Type II diabetes. Avandia is widely prescribed in the UK but its efficacy has been challenged in the USA on the basis of an apparent increase in heart attacks amongst users. In order to resolve the debate, the Mayo clinic, an American research organization not dependent on commercial funding, analyzed more than 200 studies of the drug published in respectable journals. It revealed that 87 per cent of the authors whose papers reported positively on Avandia had financial links with GlaxoSmithKline, the company that markets the drug. The Mayo researchers concluded that the debate around Avandia is being perpetuated in the face of clear evidence that the drug does increase the risk of heart attack, by scientists with financial conflicts of interest which render them non-objective in their views (Laurence, 2010: 8).

The women in this book were research-aware. They knew that the evidence can say whatever the authorities citing it wish it to say, and secondly, that the evidence is only as good as the stage the research has reached (or as the amount of funding allocated to pursue a particular field of enquiry). They noted that women who gave birth in hospital often laboured in bed and spent second stage on their backs. Yet they knew, without necessarily being able to cite *Effective Care in Pregnancy and Childbirth* (Enkin *et al.* 2000) that this is unhelpful to labouring women. One of the reasons they chose home birth was for the freedom it would give them to labour in whatever position felt right to them. When presented with an apparently illogical point of view, such as its being unsafe to labour at home if you are HIV positive, Leonie searched the internet to find the evidence. She couldn't find any. The women did find evidence, however, that being frightened affects the progress of labour – evidence that never figured in their conversations with health professionals. In other words, they discovered for themselves the phenomenon that the anthropologist, Brigitte Jordan, famously described in 1977: namely that there is knowledge and then there is 'authoritative knowledge'. Commenting on this, Rapp noted in 1992:

> Authoritative knowledge isn't produced by access to complex technology, or some will to hierarchy in the abstract. It is a way of organizing power relations in a room which makes them seem literally unthinkable in any other way.

A story told to me as I was researching this book illustrates the consciousness among at least some obstetricians of owning authoritative knowledge. The woman whose story it is was 37 years old, expecting her first child and requesting a home birth. She had a BMI of 34. A routine appointment with her consultant went as follows:

Consultant: Do you seriously want to go ahead and risk your baby's life on this utterly ridiculous idea? And what does your husband think about it? It's his baby, too!
Woman: He's quite happy with it and so is my midwife.
Consultant: Well, I'm not a midwife; I'm an obstetrician, so I know!

The knowledge the women in this book held because of their lived experience as childbearing women was considered merely to be 'knowledge'; the knowledge possessed by the health professionals whom they encountered was '*authoritative* knowledge'.

More humility in relation to 'the evidence' and more insight into the psychological sequelae of labelling women as 'high-risk' might lead to a more democratic and humane maternity service. Despite their courage and conviction, the women in this book were not immune to the effects of having a 'high-risk' label attached to them. This extract from Margret's story demonstrates how prophecies can easily become self-fulfilling. Remember that Margret had had three large babies and had been repeatedly told that she ran a serious risk of shoulder dystocia:

> I got to second stage and I didn't realize how much of an effect the last few weeks had had on my mental health around birth. I knew the way they had been measuring me wasn't a good way and was really variable depending on who was doing the measuring. I knew all that. I knew that the chances of everything being fine with this baby were great because I'd previously given birth to a 10lbs baby in very unfavourable circumstances, lying flat on my back. I knew I was doing everything to minimize my risk of shoulder dystocia. I was in a good position; I was in the birth pool. I'd done everything I could. But at that point, I got really really

scared and I said, 'I think the baby's stuck; the baby's not coming out; the baby's stuck; I can't get it out'. And I said to my midwife, 'There's something holding me back; I can't push this baby out. I can't do it; I'm just too scared that the baby is going to get stuck'.

And both of the midwives there spoke to me and said, 'It's understandable that you are going to feel like this, Margret, after what you have been through, but you are doing it; you're doing absolutely fine' and they talked me through it and they reassured me and they were saying, 'You're doing fantastic. You wouldn't have got to this point in your labour if the baby was that big; you are doing fine', and they reassured me and mothered me and helped me through it. Eventually, they'd built my confidence to such a point that I said, 'Yes, I can do it, can't I?' And my body just took over.

Then I got to another point where I said to them, 'I know you're going to say my baby will be here in a moment because you've heard women make these noises before, but it's not going to work for me'. They said, 'Of course it's going to work for you, Margret!' And he was born in the water a few moments later.

Owing to the unstinting support she received from her independent midwife and midwife friend, Margret was able to escape the vicious cycle in which risk labelling so often traps women.

The same vicious cycle traps midwifery and obstetric professionals:

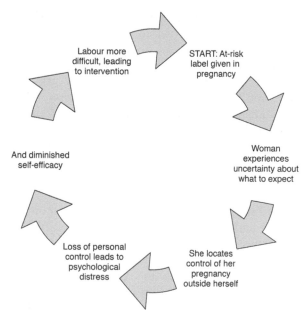

Figure 3.2
Based on Jordan's and Murphy's article, 2009.

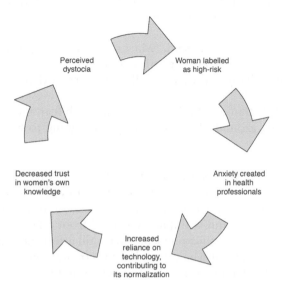

Figure 3.3

In many of the women's stories, the fear in the health professionals caring for them is almost palpable. Doctors and midwives are naturally as subject to contemporary childbirth mythology as are the women whom they serve. An article in the *British Journal of Midwifery* quotes a home birth mother as saying that 'fear and panic had been emanating from the midwife, despite her saying that she was experienced at caring for women at home' (Hall 1999: 223). A lack of midwifery faith in physiological birth, compounded by institutional pressure to subscribe to a medical model of care has been described elsewhere (e.g. Houghton and Lavender 2008; Walton *et al.* 2005), raising serious questions about the future of normal birth, of which midwives are the guardians.

Midwives' fear is as multi-faceted as is childbearing women's. Increasing lack of experience of uninterfered-with birth may render them as unfamiliar with how to assist birth without technology as are doctors. It is not uncommon now for student midwives to complete their degree-level training without ever having seen a straightforward vaginal birth on the labour ward, or even having seen birth without epidural analgesia. Fear of their own hierarchy, of longitudinal and horizontal bullying, have been recorded by Deery and Kirkham (2006). The health service itself appears to have surveillance at its core, with its rhetoric of providing individualized care at serious odds with its insistence that employees should stick rigidly to policies and protocols. Nearly a decade ago, Kirkham *et al.* (2002) wrote of an increasing sense that the maternity service was 'controlled by rules and constantly inspected'. There is no reason to think this has changed.

Midwives' fear is evident in the women's stories. Margret described an appointment with the midwife at her GP's surgery:

> She was lovely and she said, 'Margret, I am going to tell you this in confidence . . . everyone is terrified that you are going to have this 11 or 12 pound baby and they are all very worried that they will have to be your midwife'.
>
> And I was thinking that if there's this much fear and all that adrenaline floating around, there is no way I am going to be able to labour effectively.

In this case, the midwife is prepared to state openly that her colleagues are afraid, and the mother instantly understands how this will affect her. As Michel Odent has commented on numerous lecture tours, adrenaline is a contagious hormone, and will quickly spread from one person to another. Even if midwives' fear is unexpressed, it will still affect the course of labour. The midwives' anxiety at Mia's birth led to intrusive behaviour that necessitated the mother having to be assertive while simultaneously coping with her labour:

> We called the midwives. One came and wanted to do an internal as soon as she got here and I said, 'I don't really want one' and she said, 'Well, we need to find out where you're at'. And she asked me about three times pretty close in succession whether she could just do 'a little internal' and I said, 'No, not really'. Eventually my friend stepped in and said, 'She's been very clear with you, and she doesn't want an internal; you are just going to have to trust her'.
>
> However, she kept asking me and I remember leaning over the sofa bed at one point and she said, 'Could I just, you know, do an internal now, in the position that you're happy with' and I said, 'I don't want you to do it' and she just would not leave me alone. So I was having to be really assertive while in labour.

Erin's request for a home birth met with a response from her midwife that was so out of proportion to the modest caution that might reasonably have been expected in the case of a mother who had previously lost a baby, not as a result of labour complications but because of a rare genetic condition, that it seems likely to have been generated purely by fear:

> Me and my husband were really excited and were in no doubt that we wanted a home birth. It felt really positive and so I mentioned it to my midwife the following day just as I was having my blood pressure taken and she promptly told me that I wouldn't be allowed to have a home birth until I'd had at least one baby vaginally in hospital. And she said, 'I wouldn't want to be your midwife and I certainly won't come to your

house. Look, I'm retiring in two years and I don't want this on my record
to ruin my career when it all goes tits up'.

The response from this particular woman was not the compliance that the
midwife's comments were intended to produce but, unfortunately, quite the
reverse:

So I contacted AIMS and read up on all the NICE guidelines.

It is an irony for the health service that risk management strategies very often
create not gratitude on the part of clients, but resentment and a tendency for
them to turn to the law when things go wrong – a course of action which the
NHS is hugely dedicated to preventing. As is often the case in human affairs,
actions taken to achieve a certain end may achieve quite the opposite; in the
case of risk management, this is because it is not, as it claims to be, rational
and systematic, but rather, as Walsh observes, 'biased to certain values and
politically motivated' (p. 474).

Labelling people according to perceived risk creates expectations in patients
that, having identified problems, health professionals will be able to do
something about them and achieve positive outcomes. Health professionals working in maternity care are acutely aware that obstetric cases are the
most costly in medical litigation, with, for example, one third of the NHS
compensation bill for London accounted for by payouts to women treated on
obstetric wards (Widdup and Goodchild 2009). High-risk labelling may be
intended to describe the patient's condition, but it also describes the perceived
risk to the doctor. To control this risk for both parties, the maximum level
of intervention may be employed, with each intervention steadily increasing the original risk even as it attempts to control it. If outcomes are less
than favourable, or tragedies occur, expectations are disappointed, distress
and resentment are generated and people hit back through complaints and
litigation. Another vicious cycle is in operation (see Figure 3.4).

In general, women's choices are constrained by their not surprising tendency to assess their own risk according to their health professional carers'
assessment of it (Jordan and Murphy 2009). What is remarkable, almost
iconoclastic, about the women whose stories are told in this book, is that they
were prepared to take the responsibility for assessing their risk themselves.
The various influences which led them to decide that they were not at risk,
or that the risk to their own and their babies' well-being would be greater in
hospital than it would be at home, were, they felt, as legitimate as the influences that health professionals brought, knowingly or unknowingly, to bear
on their own assessments.

The logical outcome of labelling nearly everyone as at some kind of risk
is to create a nation of 'worried well', diminishing enjoyment in the good
health that the wealthier people of the world are, in fact, privileged to enjoy,
and draining the health service of resources for those who are genuinely in

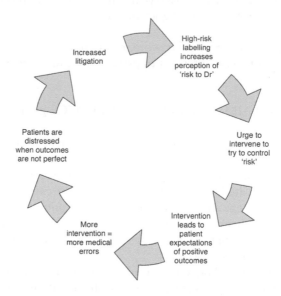

Figure 3.4

need of care and treatment. In 1984, Osada wrote:

> Defects in public health education and the irresponsible or sometimes sensational medical information released by the mass media are causing an excessive increase in the population's demand for health care services. As a result, so-called 'worried well' patients are increasing and health care institutions are crowded with such patients who play a major role in increasing national medical spending.
>
> (p. 359)

While this article was probably ahead of its time in drawing attention to the disastrous effects of undermining people's ability to read their own bodies, it is interesting that the 'blame' for the drain on resources caused by the 'worried well' is placed firmly outside the health professions themselves, on the media and 'faulty public education'. Health education is, however, very much the province of health professionals, something that has been recognized more fully in 2010 by the Self Care Campaign. This campaign was launched by a group of leading doctors, nurses and other professionals involved in primary care who are warning of the 'catastrophic impact' of the public's dependency on the NHS. The group claims that approximately £2 billion of health care money is wasted each year on adults of working age consulting their GPs for minor ailments. Their aim is to educate people to be able to differentiate between symptoms that are insignificant and those that require medical attention. The need for such education to refocus the attention of the public on health rather than on disease is the logical product of health services' tendency to concentrate on illness rather than wellness, alerting people to disasters that are very unlikely to occur (such as happened in 2009 with swine flu) and on creating a health care consumer who is 'a passive creature, dependent on professional advice' (Hewson 2004).

The maternity service, those who work in it and those who use it, are the victims of the fear that accompanies affluence – the fear of 'losing it all'. Fear generates a desire to control risk, and this is achieved by putting in place rules and regulations which become ever more stringent, and create increasing stress for those who make them, for those who implement them and for those who have to abide by them – ironically, the very people who requested them in the first place.

The women in this book were 'at risk', as measured by most risk-assessment tools used in NHS Trusts. Their insistence on having a home birth 'against medical advice' challenged the validity of those tools and the whole edifice of risk management and fear which underpins it. An all-pervasive intolerance of risk explains the intense professional anxiety produced when the women sought to exercise choice in their childbearing decisions (Hewson 2004). They were determined to act autonomously, according to their own understanding of their situations – an understanding based on reason, emotion and trust in their bodies' ability to birth their babies. For all the rhetoric of choice in the health service and its stated commitment to recognizing and responding sensitively to the individuality of each patient, the system appeared profoundly undemocratic to the women, threatening the autonomy of both its clinicians and its patients.

Key points

- Health professionals may be as vulnerable as women to a mythology of childbirth dangers which they create from the stories they tell each other.
- The validity of risk-scoring tools used in maternity services is undetermined and such tools can mislead care decisions.
- The research evidence is always in a state of *becoming*; it is never complete.
- Providing individualized care is at odds with the onus on staff to adhere to policies and protocols.
- The logical outcome of widespread risk labelling is to create a nation of 'worried well', thereby draining the health service of resources for those who are genuinely in need.

References

Beech B. (2009) Midwifery: running down the drain. *AIMS Journal*, 21(3):5.

Campbell R. and Macfarlane A. (1994) *Where to Be Born? The Debate and the Evidence* (2nd ed.). Oxford: National Perinatal Epidemiology Unit.

Deery R. and Kirkham M. (2006) Supporting midwives to support women. In: Page L. A. and McCandlish R. (eds) *The New Midwifery: Science and sensitivity.* Edinburgh: Churchill Livingstone: 125–40.

Enkin M., Keirse M., Neilson J., Crowther C., Duley L., Hodnett E. and Hofmeyr J. (2000) *A Guide to Effective Care in Pregnancy and Childbirth* (3rd ed.). Oxford: Oxford University Press.

Furedi F. (2006) *Culture of Fear* (2nd ed.). London: Continuum International Publishing Group.

Hall J. (1999) Home birth: the midwife effect. *British Journal of Midwifery,* 7(4):223–7.

Hewson B. (2004) Risk aversion and the culture of fear. *British Journal of Midwifery,* 12(1):5.

Houghton G. and Lavender T. (2008) Factors influencing choice in birth place: an exploration of the views of women, their partners and professionals. *Evidence Based Midwifery,* June, available online at www.rcm.org.uk (accessed 17 March 2010).

Jordan B. (1977) The self diagnosis of early pregnancy: an investigation of lay competence. *Medical Anthropology,* 1(2):1–38.

Jordan R. G. and Murphy P. A. (2009) Risk assessment and risk distortion: finding the balance. *Journal of Midwifery and Women's Health,* 54(3):191–200.

Kingdon C., Lavender T., Gyte G., Cattrell R., Singleton V. and Neilson J. (2003) Who's choosing caesarean section? *British Journal of Midwifery,* 11(6):391.

Kirkham M., Stapleton H., Thomas G. and Curtis P. (2002) Checking, not listening: how midwives cope. *British Journal of Midwifery,* 10(7):447–50.

Koster O. (2001) One in six women too terrified to give birth. *Daily Mail,* 17 December, p. 28.

Laurance J. (2010) Glaxo funded backers of 'danger' drug. *International Independent,* 19 March.

Merialdi M. (2010) 'Women create life'. International Conference on Birth and Primal Health, Gran Canaria, 28 February.

Montgomery T. (1958) Physiologic considerations in labor and the puerperium. *American Journal of Obstetrics and Gynecology,* October.

Osada H. (1984) The Structure of health care service – so-called worried well patients and psychosomatic medicine. *J OUEH* 6 (4):359–68.

Rapp R. (1992) Commentary on *Birth in Twelve Cultures: Papers in honor of Brigitte Jordan,* a symposium at the annual meeting of the American Anthropological Association, December.

Royal College of Midwives (2002) *Home Birth: Position Paper 25.* London: RCM.

Royal College of Obstetricians and Gynaecologists/Royal College of Midwives (2007) *Home Births,* Joint Statement No. 2, April.

Stapleton H., Kirkham M. and Thomas G. (2002) Qualitative study of evidence-based leaflets in maternity care. *British Medical Journal,* 324:639.

Vygotsky L. S. (1978) *Mind in Society.* Cambridge: Harvard University Press.

Walsh D. (2003) Risk management is not objective. *British Journal of Midwifery,* 11(8):474.

Walton C., Yiannousiz K. and Gatsby H. (2005) Promoting midwifery-led care within an obstetric-led unit. *British Journal of Midwifery,* 13(12):750–5.

Weston R. Sharples (2005) Liberating childbirth. *AIMS Journal*, 17(3), available online at www.aims.org.uk/Journal/Vol17No3/liberatingChildbirth.htm (accessed 2 April 2010).

Widdup E. and Goodchild S. (2009) Childbirth and maternity failures cost NHS £27m a year in compensation. *London Evening Standard*, 18 August.

Websites

Evidence Based Midwifery: www.rcm.org.uk (accessed 17 March 2010).

National Childbirth Trust: www.nctpregnancyandbabycare.com/about-us/what-we-do/policy (accessed 22 March 2010).

National Health Service Litigation Authority: www.nhsla.com/home.htm (accessed 16 March 2010).

Self Care Campaign: www.selfcarecampaign.org (accessed 16 March 2010).

World Values Survey: www.worldvaluessurvey.org (accessed 17 March 2010).

4   Choice, bullying and coercion

The Royal College of Midwives published a position paper on home birth in 2002, which employed the familiar language of choice:

> It is important that the [maternity] service facilitates and promotes genuine *choice* in the location of intrapartum midwifery care.
>
> (p. 5)

Every UK government publication since *Changing Childbirth* in 1993 has insisted that choice is at the heart of the maternity service, that it is the right of every childbearing woman and the goal of every NHS Trust. Nevertheless, ten years later, overuse of the rhetoric had largely devalued the phrase 'informed choice', and McCourt *et al.* (2004) stated:

> Little is known about what constitutes informed choice.
>
> (p. 414)

Originally the mantra of the retail industry, where providing customers with a 'choice' of goods was, and remains, the way to maximize profits, 'choice' became a by-word in health care when Margaret Thatcher introduced the concept of the internal market in a vain attempt to control the escalating cost of the NHS. It is, however, far clearer as to what choice means in terms of choosing a car or selecting a holiday than when applied to health care when the choices patients make may affect the rest of their lives.

While most people today are fairly sophisticated shoppers and are aware of the ways in which supermarkets, for example, manipulate their choices through advertising, location of products in their stores, special offers and free parking, they are far less clear about how their health care choices might be influenced by the professionals who provide them. The professionals themselves may be unaware that they have the potential to manipulate patients' choice or may consider doing so justified on the basis of their superior knowledge and experience.

For informed choice to be a reality, therefore, it requires educated health care consumers and health professionals who are willing to offer it and know how to present it. The Canadian Midwifery Regulators' Consortium therefore defines 'informed choice' in terms of what it requires the midwife to *do*:

> For the midwife, this decision-making process involves taking time with the woman, listening to her questions and concerns, providing her with clear evidence-based information about the benefits and disadvantages of each choice she is considering and supporting her in her decision-making.

The centrality of choice in the consciousness of both health care consumers and of health professionals has motivated continuing attempts to pin down exactly what it means. Coleman (2004) explored choice from the point of view of the childbirth educator and how she can assist parents attending antenatal classes to make decisions about the care that is best for them. She argued that 'informed choice' must be underpinned by 'freedom' and 'knowledge' and by the reality of there being 'alternatives' to choose among. In a more recent analysis, Law *et al.* (2009) considered that:

> When choice is 'informed' it is based on the possession and understanding of information and reflects the values of the decision-maker.
>
> (p. 311)

This is an uncomfortable definition for many health care staff. While putting information into the possession of patients does not necessarily have to mean a shift of control away from professionals, as soon as patients are allowed to apply their 'own values' to how they interpret and use the information they now possess, control moves into their territory. Patients' 'values' may be entirely at odds with health professionals'; indeed, they may be at odds with those of most other people. Nevertheless, according to Law *et al.* (2009) and to the NHS, they are an essential part of each individual's decision-making and an inalienable element of 'informed choice':

> Good communication is essential, supported by evidence based information, to allow women to reach informed decisions about their care. The views, beliefs and values of the woman, her partner and her family in relation to her care and that of her baby should be sought and respected at all times.
>
> (NICE 2007: 2)

The way in which health services respond when people do apply their own values to information is the most fascinating aspect of the stories of the women in this book.

If having information is the first step to making an informed choice, how knowledgeable were the women who decided to choose home birth against medical and midwifery advice? Every woman in this book had researched her situation extensively, sometimes because she could not get information about it from her health carers. Nor did the women deliberately avoid looking at information that was unsettling and could be seen as supporting a choice different from the one they wanted to make. Maria-Sofie tested positive for group B strep at 32 weeks of pregnancy and was informed that this prevented her from choosing a home birth because she would need to receive antibiotics in labour, and these could only be given at the hospital. She took a rigorous approach to researching her situation, consulting first with her independent midwife and then on the internet where she found some reassuring and some very unsettling material:

> I searched on the internet. I found out that the chances of passing the infection to your baby are really very small. However, when you do searches on the internet, you come across some awful pictures of dead babies and it starts you thinking. I just couldn't cope if that was me.

At this point, she had a good knowledge of the risks posed by group B strep, and she was also very clear in her own mind that nothing was more important than protecting her baby from harm, and herself from experiencing a birth tragedy. She both knew the facts and understood what they meant for her. Since she had not being given choices, she proceeded to work them out for herself:

> I decided that my choices were either to go to hospital and have antibiotics, or to stay at home and not have any antibiotics, or to explore the route of having the antibiotics at home.

She then took the responsibility of approaching her GP to ask her to prescribe antibiotics for the midwife to administer at home. The GP gave her some more information of which she had not previously been aware, namely that there was a possibility of anaphylactic shock associated with administration of antibiotics. Far from ignoring this new information, Maria-Sofie then set up a meeting between the GP and her independent midwife in order that the health professionals might consider whether this was truly an obstacle to a home birth. Following the meeting, the GP agreed to prescribe adrenaline along with the antibiotics for use at home.

Finally, all three adults exercised their freedom to make choices based on high quality information, professional expertise and personal values. The process of informed decision-making was, however, driven in this case by the mother with a very noticeable shift of power from professional to health care consumer. It is this which makes the story so unusual – some might say shocking.

Just as 'informed choice' is both difficult to understand and difficult to implement, so patient empowerment is equally so. Maria-Sofie took the initiative in her own care; what would happen if all patients did the same? Is it realistic to allow patients to determine their own care to such an extent?

These are questions that need answering if the rhetoric of informed choice and patient empowerment is to have any integrity.

Lili's experience was different; she was expecting her first baby and tried hard to obtain information from her midwife, but was blocked:

> [At the booking appointment] I said to her, 'What are my options for where I could have the baby?' And she said, 'You'll be booked into St. G's', and I said, 'I thought perhaps of a home birth?' She said, 'No, you can't have a home birth' and I said, 'Oh, OK, why is that?' And she said, 'Because of where you live'. So she said there was no way I could have a home birth.

Lili continued to attend her antenatal appointments, and raised the issue of a home birth again, to be met with neither a change in the midwife's attitude, nor any further information as to why a home birth on an island in the Thames was impossible. Thrown on her own resources, Lili consulted a woman experienced in birthing, namely her sister who had had four babies, and she suggested consulting an independent midwife. This was a choice that Lili did not see as immediately desirable because:

> I'm very pro the NHS and so was a bit taken aback by the suggestion.

She reflected and decided that she could at least talk to an independent midwife; as a result of this conversation, she made her choice to meet the midwife's fee so that she could have her home birth. Her reasoning was as follows:

> I couldn't have a home birth on the NHS.
> I knew quite a few people who had had awful birth experiences and this had impacted on their ability to bond with their babies.
> It struck me that people who had had good birth experiences got on better in dealing with motherhood.

She had carefully observed and analyzed the early parenting experiences of friends, and in order to protect her relationship with her baby, undertook research which enabled her to identify a previously unidentified choice, namely to employ an independent midwife. In Lili's case, her choice depended on her ability to take the initiative, the strength of her personal values *and* the financial resources to pay for private health care. Where Maria-Sofie was able to achieve patient empowerment by negotiation with health care staff within the NHS, Lili's informed decision-making took her outside the health service into the private sector.

Alessia's efforts to exercise choice in an adult manner, respecting the intelligence and integrity of the professionals with whom she came into contact, resulted in three months of increasingly unpleasant interviews with senior staff. A home birth had been agreed at the start of her pregnancy prior to a scan which revealed that she was expecting twins who would be her fifth and sixth babies. Following this,

> The midwife's immediate reaction was, 'Oh you can't possibly have a home birth; that's out now' and I said, 'Why?' And she said, 'There are far too many complications; you can't possibly even dream of that'.

Alessia returned home to research twin birth on the internet, to consult with eminent midwives such as Mary Cronk, to talk to other health professionals and to discuss the situation at length with her partner. She decided that a home birth was still right for her. She therefore wrote to the Head of Midwifery at the local hospital and was invited to a meeting:

> The Head of Midwives sat with her Supervisor of Midwives and the discussion was based on risks, and especially postpartum haemorrhage and it was a very sombre meeting, a very serious meeting, lots of raised eyebrows, lots of sombre faces and frowns.

> Alessia and her husband felt: like children who were doing something that was very, very naughty, like bungee jumping off a cliff or something very irresponsible.

This was a common theme in the women's stories. Lili commented that in all her encounters with health professionals during the first half of her pregnancy:

> I felt like I was always in trouble for something.

Adults can impose their will on children because there is an imbalance of power between the two. At some point in their efforts to gain permission for a home birth, the women in this book were always brought into contact with a senior health professional who tried to exert a parental type of authority, doubtless in the interests of protecting the mother from making an unsafe choice. This behaviour begs the question of whether informed choice can be exercised in the face of oppressive authority, and whether exercising authority in order to obtain compliance is appropriate. It has been argued that not only is it appropriate, it is the responsibility of health professionals to exercise power:

> It is absurd to say that there is no truth defined by experts, that patients are equals, or to allow patients to define conditions and treatment . . . Clinical effectiveness depends on understanding the patient's beliefs and expectations. Patients are, however, not equals, and their beliefs do not have the ontological status of medical knowledge.

Denial of the status of doctors and of medicine's tradition of research is false democracy.

(McQueen 2002)

There is a debate to be had here. What is probably not debatable is that bullying is never justified in the attempt to get patients to bow to superior wisdom. Olweus, the Swedish psychologist, considered to be the father of bully and victim research, states:

> A person is bullied when he or she is exposed, repeatedly and over time, to negative actions on the part of one or more other persons, and he or she has difficulty defending himself or herself.

There was a recurrent pattern in the way in which pressure to accept a hospital birth was brought to bear on the women in this book, a pattern which fits the description of bullying given above. Pressure was exerted at a time when the women had difficulty in defending themselves, namely as they were approaching the end of pregnancy, when they were tired and emotional, and should have been preparing quietly, both physically and mentally, for the arrival of their babies. It was at this stage that local midwives, unable to get the women to see their point of view, referred the women up the hierarchy to continue the debate. Mette was asked to see the Supervisor of Midwives when she was 'heavily pregnant, tired, very emotional'. She had to take her two-year-old toddler with her to a meeting that was scheduled for 3pm at the hospital, an environment she finds frightening. The supervisor arrived three hours late:

> She didn't actually get in until 6 o'clock, so I was waiting in the hospital with my child, feeling very tired, for about three and a half hours. I don't like hospitals at the best of times, but I didn't mind. I think I minded when her first words to me were, 'I have no agenda'.

The mother felt that, on the contrary, the senior person very definitely did have an agenda; why else had this special meeting been arranged? The imbalance of power which is the basis for bullying became quickly apparent to her:

> It just felt like I was there by myself. I think that when you are pregnant and emotional, you are very volatile and vulnerable; you really need someone there with you and I felt like I was being shouted at. I know they weren't meaning to do that. However, the supervisor's manner was quite aggressive and upfront even though she said she had 'no agenda'. She read through my birth plan and nit picked it, and mentioned within about ten minutes of the start of our conversation – death of the baby, brain damage of the baby, death of the mother (me!) and all of this when I'm tired and have been hanging around the hospital for nearly four hours.

The mother is reduced to tears which, is taken as proof that she is not thinking clearly:

> I thought, 'I just can't take any more' and I burst into tears and obviously, she thought, 'Oh, ho – she's not coping!'

Mette took the only action she could to preserve her dignity and her mental health. She retreated:

> I said, 'I am not going to talk about this any more because you are not encouraging me; you are just trying to pressurize me to come into hospital even though you say you have no agenda'.

The effects of bullying are documented by Olweus as depression, low self-esteem, health problems and suicidal thoughts (www.olweus.org). The bullying Mia endured drove her to the brink of desperation, as we will see later in this chapter. She was given an appointment to see the consultant when she asked for a home birth with her third child after two previous births of large babies. Although she tried to explain that:

> I felt I knew my body very well and that I felt my body wasn't going to produce a baby that was too big for my hips and for my birth canal,

there was no attempt at dialogue on the consultant's part, but merely a statement of her authority:

> Your babies are too big and you'll get shoulder dystocia and there is absolutely no way I would give my consent to a home birth.

It is characteristic of bullying that the target (victim) attempts to present her case in a reasonable manner, but achieves nothing because the reason that she is being bullied is precisely because she is reasonable. It is not the target's rationale for her actions that provokes the attack, but her competence, coupled with her vulnerability. This is not to say that any of the health professionals whom the women encountered were bullies or would have been considered by colleagues as bullies; however, they do appear to have been the agents of a bullying maternity service that disliked clients who were tall poppies and was determined to cut them down to size.

If asked whether they considered the kind of behaviour described by Mette and Mia as acceptable, professionals might well respond that the behaviour of the senior personnel involved was not aggressive but simply assertive. However assertive behaviour is based on respect for the other person, recognition that the values of both parties deserve consideration, discussion which does not invoke blame on either side, and the anticipation of a compromise which might not be entirely satisfactory but will leave both parties with their self-esteem intact. Nor does assertiveness carry with it a threat that there will be negative consequences for the other party should she fail to submit to the arguments and proposals put before her.

People who become the focus of bullying are pre-eminently not *victims*; they are targeted precisely because they have a mature outlook, have reflected upon their circumstances and their choices, can articulate these convincingly and are calmly sure of themselves. Such people have a strong sense of their value as intelligent human beings. They do not rely on others to make their decisions for them; they are active rather than passive in their lives and they respect authority when it presents itself reasonably and caringly.

Bullying is very rarely an isolated incident; in fact, it is characterized by the fact that it is repeated. Mia left the consultation with her consultant feeling 'absolutely floored'. This was not to be the final encounter with medical authority, however. Five days later, she received a letter:

> She [the consultant] had photocopied a chapter out of an obstetric textbook on shoulder dystocia. A lot of textbooks start with a quote from older texts, don't they? And this chapter did; there was a quote at the head of the chapter in very small writing, and it described how one mother's labour had ended in the death of a baby from shoulder dystocia, and the final words were 'and the poor soul lay there lifeless'. That's what she sent me. It was horrendous.

Mia was six months pregnant when she received this, and the effect on her was devastating:

> This might sound like I was insane, but I thought the only thing I could do was to have an abortion; that's what I thought. I felt trapped in the pregnancy. I thought, 'I can't go through a hospital birth again, I won't do it, I can't contemplate going through that again'. It was a nightmare and the pregnancy was there and how could I end it?

In one of a series of articles exploring whether there is any substance to the notion of 'informed choice', Stapleton *et al.* (2002) recognized that both midwives and obstetricians, when confronted by women who want to make choices which are inconvenient, unpopular or 'not allowed' in their units, will resort to 'shroud–waving' in an attempt to force the women to conform. A further strategy was simply not to listen to the women and to avoid having conversations with them by substituting form-filling instead. This appears to be what happened in Mia's case, where the consultant chose to threaten her via a written communication following the unsatisfactory face to face encounter.

At this point in her story, Mia found herself with two choices, both of which risked her mental health. Either she could continue to choose a home birth and face ongoing pressure to conform to the consultant's wishes, pressure which she was now finding intolerable, or she could decide to go into hospital which was charged with memories of her two previous frightening and painful births. She made her choice for home birth, based on her own assessment of how best to remain sane:

> I reckoned I would absolutely have preferred to hide under a bush on a common plot out there to give birth than go anywhere near the hospital. This is actually a rational feeling because the risks to your mental state, to your emotions of going through such a traumatic thing again, are potentially catastrophic, so the risks of whatever they think could go wrong under that bush are relative, you know, and not so bad.

The harmful effects of bullying are well known and accepted. Children who are targeted at school perform badly in examinations, become withdrawn, stop communicating with their parents, and may, on tragic occasions, harm or even kill themselves. Depression and anxiety are common among adults; people who were once competent to handle their own lives become incompetent and dependent. The following extract from Bully Online sums up how the maternity service appeared to the women who were its clients:

> Bullies exhibit plausibility, certitude, self-assuredness, untouchability, a sense of invulnerability and an unerring belief in their rightness and infallibility.

Mette, Mia and the other women were unusual in the resistance they mounted to the heavy-handed attempts to dominate them. That is why they are interesting – because their unusual behaviour elicited responses apparently inherent in the health service but which are usually not seen because, by and large, there is very little need to bully women into conforming. They are quite willing to toe the line. Women conform because they trust their health professional carers to know best, and always to have their best interests at heart (Stapleton *et al.*, 2002a). They live in a culture where, despite some knocks to medical supremacy, the consultant and whoever represents him or her (and this includes in popular thought, midwives and nurses) remain immensely respected and trusted. Questioning is considered either inappropriate, impertinent or demanding more courage than most of us have. Women do not threaten the system because they are vulnerable in pregnancy, and because they do not think that birth can be better than it is, even if it doesn't appear to be very satisfactory as it is currently managed:

> Where [women] express a preference, it is generally for whatever arrangements they have experienced, rather than for other possible arrangements . . . women's expectations of maternity care are very low and . . . 'not minding' certain treatments means very little.
>
> (Porter and MacIntyre 1984: 1200)

The drive to get dissenting women to conform to Trust policies turned midwives and consultants into bullies and occasionally led them to give mis-information in order to strengthen their hand. A disturbing example of this occurred in Maria-Sofie's story in relation to a midwife appointment that had no immediate reference to her decision to have a home birth:

> The community midwife told me that I needed to have blood tests and one of these was HIV. I said I didn't need that one because I had had all the blood tests with my first pregnancy and they had been absolutely fine, so she could test for anaemia and things like that, but I told her that she didn't need to test for HIV because I hadn't got it. She said, 'Well, we still like to test anyway' and I said, 'But you don't need to because I haven't got it; I didn't have it last time' and she said, 'Well, things change' and insinuated that my partner might have been having an affair. I assured her that he hadn't and then she told me that I might have caught HIV on holiday from a swimming pool.

When HIV first hit the news in the 1980s, understanding of the disease by most health professionals was limited, and by the media and general public even more so. This led to widespread panic that HIV might be caught from any surface previously touched by someone infected with the virus. A series of advertisements, such as the one depicting a mug and the slogan, 'You must be a mug to think you can catch HIV from this' attempted to reassure people that this was not the case.

Misinformation about HIV persists, however, making it difficult to reduce the stigma attached to those who are living with the infection. To add to this misinformation, deliberately, can only be considered unethical. If Maria-Sofie's midwife did not know that HIV cannot be caught from a swimming pool, there is something wrong with her training; if she did know, there is something wrong with her understanding of her code of professional conduct. Such incidents are highly detrimental to the image and authority of the midwifery profession and add fuel to the fires of those who feel that it is not, in any case, serving women well:

> Unfortunately, it is not enough to know what your rights are; you also have to know how to deal with the lies, ignorance or misinformation handed out with total confidence by some professionals who ought to know better.
>
> (Beech 2005)

Reports of midwives manipulating information to ensure compliance with Trust policies have appeared in the midwifery literature elsewhere. Hindley's and Thomson's study (2005) of electronic foetal monitoring described how the need to actively manage labouring women in accordance with medical dictates led midwives to interact with them in a dishonest manner. What drove the midwife to suggest to Maria-Sofie that she could catch HIV from a swimming pool is hard to imagine – perhaps it was an unconsidered backlash against a client challenging her authority; perhaps it was simply one woman's irritation at being thwarted by another; perhaps it was desperation to tick all the boxes on the Trust's forms. Whatever the reason, if it was designed to exact conformity, it had the opposite effect:

> I said, 'I don't think you can catch HIV like that', and then she told me that if I didn't agree to the blood test, I would jeopardise my chances of having a home birth, at which point I informed her that it was her duty of care to come out to me whether I had HIV or not, and I didn't, but it was still my choice not to have the test.
> So that's when I decided I was definitely going to have an independent midwife.

Perhaps the heaviest handed strategy disclosed in the women's stories to attempt to coerce them into having their babies in hospital was to threaten them with the very thing that health professionals are so frightened of themselves: namely, the sanction of the law. Interestingly, despite the fact that the current generation of childbearing women are the daughters and grand-daughters of women who experienced the social liberation of the 1960s, and then lived through the Thatcher years when the right of the individual to self determination was considered absolute, one of the most frequently asked questions at antenatal classes is, 'Can I refuse treatments once I am in hospital?' The belief persists that by virtue of walking through the doors of the hospital, the patient has given her tacit consent to whatever procedures the hospital staff feel appropriate in her case. Indeed, such an assumption might have been justified less than 50 years ago. Beverley Beech, Honorary President of the Association for Improvements in the Maternity Services, notes that her own hospital notes from the 1970s contained the following statement inside the front cover:

> The [Medical Defence] Union does not consider that a maternity patient need give her written consent to any operative or manipulative procedures that are normally associated with childbirth. When she enters hospital for her confinement it can be assumed that she assents to any necessary procedure including the administration of local or general anesthetic.
> (Beech 2005)

Expectant parents today still wonder whether they can be forced to follow medical advice. Following the refusal by her GP, HIV consultant and obstetric specialist even to consider her having a home birth, Leonie and her husband made an expensive appointment with a lawyer (one they could not easily afford) to find out if they could be forced to have their baby in hospital. Lack of understanding of the legal position among both women and professionals is evident from the stories the women told of their mission to achieve a home birth. Hospitals were very prepared to threaten legal measures to enforce their policies and women were unsure of their ground. Margret was visited by the Supervisor of Midwives when she was 38 weeks, and was handed a document written on Trust-headed notepaper:

> This is a disclosure to say if anything happens at home, you take full responsibility and that you will transfer into hospital if we deem it necessary.

Such a 'disclosure' has, of course, no force at all in law. The mother can and should assume responsibility for her choices; midwives and doctors, however, are not exempt from practising competently under whatever circumstances the woman's choices oblige them to work. If they feel that the woman's choices are risky, they must inform her of the problems they foresee, but should those problems materialize, they remain responsible for the actions they take and can be judged on the basis of the standards of a responsible body of midwifery opinion. Should their actions reach those standards, they cannot be accused of negligence (Bolam Test).

Margret was unsure of the legal implications of the document she was being asked to sign; she was, however, quick to spot the loophole that it might provide for staff to get her to come into hospital for the birth of her baby:

> I said, 'What do you mean by 'deem necessary'? I am going to agree to transfer into hospital – for what reasons? Can you give me some examples?' And she said, 'Well, if we deem it necessary'. I said, 'But you 'deem' a hospital birth necessary right now, so are you going to turn up and immediately say I've got to go into hospital?'

After taking a night to consider, Margret refused to sign the paper. Alessia was also presented with an 'Action Plan' following several acrimonious meetings with the Head of Midwifery; this was a five-page document, which:

> Stated that we were totally responsible legally for anything that happened at home and that if anything went wrong, it would be our fault and we would be liable and it would have nothing to do with them.

It appears that the authority of the law was being invoked in these quasi-legal documents to frighten the women into agreeing to have their babies in hospital. Informed choice now becomes a legal battlefield and the mother's right to choose where she gives birth is felt by Trusts to be contestable in law. Were this the case (which it is not), it is possible to envisage situations where police cars are arriving at the home of a woman suspected of labouring with a 'big baby' or under any other medically determined unfavourable circumstances, to remove her by force to the nearest maternity unit.

It is likely that all of the health professionals involved in the care of the women in this book would be shocked to find that their actions might be interpreted as bullying. Doubtless they considered that the strenuous efforts they made to persuade the mothers to give up their plans for home birth were, in fact, 'going the extra mile' in terms of fulfilling their duty of care, and were motivated by the strong desire to protect both mother and child. And yet, their actions and the effects of those actions on the mothers' well-being are certainly akin to the emotional bullying that characterizes toxic workplace relationships and domestic abuse situations which we have no hesitation in describing as bullying. Perhaps the fact that none of these professionals would see their actions in this way is the most worrying aspect of the stories the women told. Behaviour that would not be condoned in other relationships appears to have been acceptable when trying to obtain consent to an intervention considered medically appropriate.

The women's stories reveal considerable lack of clarity in the health service about the limits of patients' right to choose, about the point at which it is reasonable and perhaps obligatory for health professionals to constrain those choices, and whether the law has any part to play in bringing about conformity to professional advice.

Midwives themselves are not without experience of being bullied both as students and as qualified practitioners. Writing about her reasons for quitting the profession, this midwife posted the following on a midwifery website:

> One of my articles provoked the wrath of the local midwifery hierarchy as I had dared to criticise the culture of midwifery I was witnessing as a student on labour ward. This was the first time I was 'brought into the office' – a little bit of pressure, a hint of bullying, and I wasn't conforming.
>
> (Walcott 2010)

Another told me:

> I was not supposed to challenge the status quo, nor was I supposed to question the many changes handed down from above. If I did, it landed me in hotter water and nobody really wanted to listen anyway. It was easier to roll over and say nothing.
>
> (private communication)

One of the papers arising from the informed choice study conducted by Stapleton *et al.* (2002b) describes how midwives are very aware of what will happen to women who refuse to conform:

> It's unreal to encourage women to go against local policies and guidelines when we all know that if she takes that line, she'll be given a really hard time.
>
> (p. 200)

The 'really hard time' was certainly experienced by the women in this book. And to no useful end. The women did not change their point of view; nor did the health professionals. In fact, both parties became more deeply entrenched in their beliefs about what was the right course of action. Finally, all the babies were born at home as the women intended and all were born safely. One of the babies was born before the midwife could arrive – partly the result of the woman's partner calling the hospital late in her labour and partly the result of the Trust's insistence that only a senior midwife could attend the birth and being unable to find one when needed. It is hard to understand how the safety of the women's births was improved by the unpleasant meetings that took place in late pregnancy between them and senior health professionals, or how the status of the medical or midwifery professions, or of the NHS, was improved by the ill feeling generated on both sides by a dispute that should have been resolved in a more 'grown-up' way.

Key points

- Patients' values may be entirely at odds with health professionals'. Nevertheless, they are an essential part of each individual's decision-making and an inalienable element of informed choice.
- Is it realistic to allow patients to determine their own care?
- The person being bullied is not targeted because of the rationale for her actions, but because she is competent and vulnerable.
- Behaviour that would not be condoned in other relationships appears to be acceptable when trying to obtain consent to an intervention considered medically appropriate.

References

Beech B. (2005) Choice: an abused concept that is past its sell-by date. *AIMS Journal*, 17(4) available online at: www.aims.org.uk/Journal/Vol17No4/Choice AbusedConcept.htm (accessed 17 February 2010).

Coleman C. (2004) Informed decision making: the benefit and risk approach. *International Journal of Childbirth Education*, 19(2):28–9.

Hindley C. and Thomson A. M. (2005) The rhetoric of informed choice: perspectives from midwives on intrapartum fetal heart rate monitoring. *Health Expectations*, 8:306–14.

Law S., Brown M. and McCalmont C. (2009) Ensuring the choice agenda is met in the maternity services. *MIDIRS Midwifery Digest*, 19(3):311–7.

McCourt C., Bick D. and Weaver J. (2004) Caesarean section: perceived demand. *British Journal of Midwifery*, 12(7):412–4.

McQueen D. (2002) Discomfort of patient power: patients are not doctors' equals. *British Medical Journal*, 324(7347):1214.

National Institute for Health and Clinical Excellence (NICE) (2007) *Intrapartum Care: Care of healthy women and their babies during childbirth*. Clinical Guideline 55. London: NICE.

Porter M. and MacIntyre S. (1984) What is, must be best: a research note on conservative or deferential responses to antenatal care provision. *Social Science and Medicine*, 19(11):1197–1200.

Royal College of Midwives (2002) *Home Birth: Position Paper 25*. London: RCM.

Stapleton H., Kirkham M., Curtis P. and Thomas G. (2002) Language used in antenatal consultations. *British Journal of Midwifery*, 10(5):273–7.

Stapleton H., Kirkham M. and Thomas G. (2002a) Qualitative study of evidence-based leaflets in maternity care. *British Medical Journal*, 324(7338):639–43.

Stapleton H., Kirkham M., Curtis P. and Thomas G. (2002b) Silence and time in antenatal care. *British Journal of Midwifery*, 10(6):393–6.

Websites

Bully Online: www.bullyonline.org (accessed 25 March 2010).

Canadian Midwifery Regulators' Consortium: http://cmrc-ccosf.ca (accessed 26 March 2010).

Olweus: bullying prevention program: www.olweus.org/public/bullying.page (accessed 26 March 2010).

Walcott L.: www.midwifery.org.uk/123lynnwalcott.htm (accessed 25 March 2010).

5   Communication and language

There seems to be a persistent belief in the public imagination, and perhaps in the professional one as well, that pregnant women are not able to think coherently. The NHS published a leaflet for expectant fathers in 2005 in which it stated:

> Pregnant women are a bit vague . . . it's their hormones. And have we mentioned the mood swings? So if she's forgotten to pay the gas bill and is reduced to tears watching 'Neighbours', don't worry, it's normal.

Indeed, the hypothesis that pregnancy affects women's memory has been of interest to researchers for a considerable time. This supposed phenomenon, labelled 'pregnesia' was the subject of a longitudinal study carried out over seven years and published recently in the *British Journal of Psychiatry* (Christensen and Mackinnon 2010). The authors concluded that: 'The hypothesis that pregnancy and motherhood are associated with persistent cognitive deterioration was not supported' (p. 126).

Pregnancy-related prejudice may be one facet of society's attitude towards women (Jarrett 2010), closely allied to the kind of prejudice encapsulated in the 'dizzy blonde' theory. This attitude is based on the supposition that women are controlled by their hormones, which over-ride their intellect, and that their reasoning is therefore impaired, especially at certain times of the month or during pregnancy. This is, however, a dangerous premise upon which to build a controlling antenatal service. Removing responsibility for their own care and that of their babies from women as they start the transition to parenthood in pregnancy is hardly an appropriate preparation for the responsibilities of being a mother. Indeed, it is the thin end of a wedge which leads to considering women as *incapable* of making their own decisions. Only a few decades ago, all decision-making was, indeed, taken away from the mother:

> Once your friends and relatives become aware of the fact that you are pregnant, you will be the recipient of all sorts of advice and suggestions from them. While this advice will be offered with the best of intentions

and from the kindliest of motives, pay no attention to it at all. No matter how many babies your Aunt Minnie had, this has no bearing on you nor does it establish her as an authority. It is often difficult not to listen, but you should politely indicate that you get your advice from your doctor.

(Goodrich 1967)

Some mothers wish to be conscious when the baby is born while others prefer to have an anesthetic. Whether or not an anesthetic is necessary and what kind of anesthetic are things your doctor will decide. Your safety and that of your baby are his responsibility. You should discuss this matter with him ahead of time so you will know what to expect.

(Department of National Health and Welfare 1970)

While this kind of patriarchy, imbued with kindly condescension, seems very dated, the debate continues to this day about whether it is appropriate for health professionals to invoke legal assistance when patients make choices that they consider dangerous. The media eagerly picks up on the more dramatic occasions when patients' choices conflict with professional advice. Such conflicts, however, occur on a daily basis over issues which are not to do with life and death. Bridget Dimond, lecturer in law, gently reminds midwifery readers:

The fact that she may be making a decision which is unwise cannot be used as evidence of incapacity.

(Dimond 2005)

Evidence of pregnancy prejudice was found in the encounters between women whose stories are told in this book and some health professionals. There was a strong tendency to treat any statement of independent thinking as puerile, and women were spoken to as if they were rebellious children who needed parental guidance. The top-down approach, generally involving the Supervisor of Midwives or Head of Midwifery, was sometimes a first line of attack in attempting to enforce compliance. Once authority was employed not in order to progress an adult-to-adult conversation, but rather to impose the will of the one over the other, satisfactory relationships between women and their carers became impossible. The work of Hunter *et al.* (2008) finds that women value two key factors in their experience of maternity care; these are the quality of the relationship with their caregivers and the amount of support they receive from them (p. 133).

It is hard to think of a word that has been more abused and misused than 'care'. Caring for someone presupposes a respectful relationship which is founded on empathy. Empathy or the ability to put oneself in the other person's shoes cannot be achieved without an intelligent engagement with what the other person is feeling, fearing and hoping for. It is an essentially intelligent virtue, not necessarily depending on education or cognitive ability, but very much depending on an emotional intelligence which is able to intuit that another person's feelings may be different from one's own, and for good reason.

An advert put out by the Birth Centre, a private midwife-run birthing facility, depicts a heavily pregnant woman and the rubric, 'You need a friend who is there for you, who understands your needs and who can guide and support both you and your partner'. Friendships are formed on a basis of equality, where each person recognizes that the other is a special human being, with a unique mixture of characteristics. Friends may agree to disagree without threatening the friendship. They can express how they feel and know that their feelings will not be judged. In the stories told by the women in this book, even mild disagreement led to a withdrawal of approval, suggesting that rhetoric about involving patients in their care as equal partners has outstripped the ability of the health service to configure itself as a democratic institution.

The consequences of treating patients like children in the health care arena is that they will behave as such, generally by doing what they are told and not questioning. This is an unhelpful role for clients to adopt when an organization is seeking to improve the service it offers; what the organization needs are clients who will tell it what they want and how it can help them to achieve their goals. The maternity service needs assertive clients who can express personal likes and preferences spontaneously, talk about how they perceive their own situation, ask for clarification rather than remain silently confused about the treatment, drugs or course of action that have been proposed, ask why health professionals are making certain suggestions and express disagreement actively when sure of their ground.

Sometimes patients will respond to attempts to treat them like children by rebelling. Rebellion can be a creative response to authority inappropriately deployed, but it may mean that both those who rebel and those who are rebelled against lose the potential to learn from each other. Half of the women in this book rebelled by removing themselves almost entirely from the maternity service by employing an independent midwife. Their relationship with these practitioners had a very different tone from that which characterized their less constructive encounters with NHS staff.

Mia, the mother of a child and pregnant for the second time, a woman in her twenties, was referred to disparagingly as a 'girl' by her consultant following an altercation regarding her wish to have a home birth:

> The consultant went out of the room and she made a phone call to my midwife and the way she was talking about me was so incredibly rude, referring to me all the time as: 'This girl'. She was really patronizing and when she walked back into the room, I said, 'I'm leaving. I'm not going to listen to you talking about me like that'. And I didn't see her again.

The effect of such disrespectful communication was that the mother decided to withdraw from both this interview and any future interviews with the consultant. The opportunity was lost for both parties to put forward their points of view, for the consultant to match her own ideas about what constitutes 'safety' in labour and birth against those of the mother's, and for the mother to benefit from the years of training and experience which had enabled the consultant to reach her senior position. Demeaning the mother by referring to her as a 'girl' was an effective way of ensuring that useful dialogue would come to an end. If women encounter criticism, impatience and negative attitudes, they naturally respond defensively and either take steps to end the encounter or, in turn, start to criticize or threaten in an attempt to regain control. At this point, the possibility of an outcome satisfactory to both parties has been lost.

Alessia was already the mother of four children when she experienced this interview regarding her request for a home birth:

> The consultant was arrogant and condescending. She spoke to me like I was a very silly little girl.
>
> [Husband] She spoke to you like you were some 16-year-old schoolgirl that had accidentally got pregnant and didn't know a thing about having a baby.
>
> Oh I got a telling off! She said, 'On your head be it, lady'. That's what she said to me.

Alessia was able to analyze very clearly the cultural expectations which underpinned the consultant's approach, a culture that one would imagine was more characteristic of the NHS sixty years ago than in the twenty-first century:

> You don't argue with the medical profession because they know what they're talking about. You don't disagree with them because they are the medical professionals and you are not. You haven't got a doctorate in medicine; they have.

Having 'authoritative knowledge' appeared to preclude the need on the consultant's part to listen respectfully to the patient's point of view, provide an impartial, unemotional and rational response, and to negotiate a compromise that might enable both parties to retain their self-respect. Instead, a series of fights ensued in which the goal on both sides became to subjugate the other.

Alessia's husband identified how the tone and underlying message of their encounters with health professionals had changed to reflect a position of dominance as his partner advanced through her pregnancy:

> The position changed from, 'We can help you if you want us to' to 'We are going to help you whether you want it or not'.

Showing by behaviour and language a lack of respect for another person's point of view is destructive of any relationship and sets up an adversarial frame of mind in the other party, encouraging them to dispute anything that is said. Maintaining two-way communication is essential for a health service which subscribes to the belief that each patient is an expert on her own 'condition' with the capacity to identify her needs and apply information shared with her to her own unique circumstances. Alessia and her husband went to the hospital to speak to health professionals on *their* territory, and then invited any members of staff who would like to witness the birth of their twins to come to *their* home. The invitation was extended also to the consultant with whom they had had such an acrimonious interview. The parents saw this as an opportunity to help staff understand what a home birth was all about and why they were so determined to have one. However, nobody from the hospital took up the invitation and the twins were born with only the two independent midwives whom the couple had employed in attendance.

A further aspect of disrespectful communication was simply to dismiss what the women were asking for as not even worthy of discussion, with the implication that any sensible adult would be able to see for herself why their requests were not reasonable.

In the following extract from Mette's and Alessia's stories, the mothers queried certain aspects of their care, and were rebutted by the midwives who took the line that any reasonable person would agree to the course of action proposed, implying thereby that the mothers' attitudes were *not* reasonable:

> I protested against being examined and having monitors as I felt it would only interrupt my concentration. And the midwives sort of said, 'Why on earth wouldn't you want to be monitored?' And they obviously thought I was being very unreasonable not to want that.
>
> Mette

> I saw her again and her immediate reaction was, 'Oh you can't possibly have a home birth; that's out now' and I said, 'Why?' And she said, 'Far too many complications'. So that was it. I'd been told I wasn't allowed to do that.
>
> Alessia

The implication of these communications appears to be either that there are areas of professional expertise which are too complex for the mother to be able to understand or that there are some situations, such as expecting twins, where choice is irrelevant and there is no value in trying to understand the perspective of the mother because it is likely to be misguided. The mother is given no information to help her understand the midwife's position. This concurs with the findings of Stapleton *et al.* (2002), who noted that information was given to women in dribs and drabs rather than in a coherent manner which would enable them to participate on an equal footing in decisions around their care. It is, of course, difficult to know how much information to give; however, Frith and Draper (2004) argue that while it might be impossible for a midwife to tell a particular woman everything she might want to know, there is presumably a bare minimum of information that is acceptable:

> [This] might be set at a level where the patient knows enough to ask questions that enable the midwife to tailor the rest of the information to the patient's needs.
>
> (p. 27)

There is no suggestion in this standard text on ethics in midwifery that it is ever acceptable to give *no* information.

This midwife not only dismissed the mother's request for a home birth but also dismissed the depth of emotion underpinning the request and the breadth of her experience of pregnancy and birth. She simply concluded, without trying to understand the mother's ideas, that she was right and the mother was wrong. However, by attempting to gain insight into why someone is choosing a particular course of action, even if disagreeing with their position, care can be more effectively tailored to the needs of the individual, leading to greater satisfaction for both professionals and clients.

The midwife's blanket refusal to consider the mother's request effectively debarred Alessia from any further participation in her own care. She was neither expected nor invited to have her own opinions. The Royal College of Midwives' position paper *Home Birth* (2002) offers practical advice on how to respond when a woman requests a home birth against midwifery advice. This paper describes the midwife's first priority as 'to sustain calm and collaborative communication' and continues by reminding practitioners that both mother and midwife share the same aims, which, though not stated, are presumably to achieve a safe and positive labour and the birth of a healthy baby. The midwife is urged to show that she respects the mother's point of view even if she does not agree with the reasoning that has brought her to her current position. It is suggested that a compromise might be reached which would involve additional back-up being provided to enable the woman to birth at home. This sensitively written directive, based both on common sense and an appreciation of the adult-to-adult relationship between the woman and her health carers, deserves to be better known and more frequently implemented.

The implications for practice of refusing outright requests for non-standard care, of dismissing a low-tech approach to care rather than a high-tech, of demonstrating emotional condescension rather than responsiveness, are considerable. In such a climate, practice becomes stagnant and reductionist, based on an assumption that one approach fits all. Expertise is lost and practice suffers. If home birth with twins is *never* 'allowed', and twins must always be born in a high-tech environment, practice becomes dependent on technology. This escalates the cost of health care, devalues practitioner skills that are independent of technology, and endangers patients in situations where the technology is not available, not maintained or inexpertly used. The assumption that certain aspects of practice can never be changed also makes a nonsense of the concept of the reflective practitioner. What is there to reflect on if nothing can ever change?

The word 'allowed' figured prominently in interviews between the women and health professionals. It is a word commonly used by parents when talking to their children, but less commonly in engagements between competent adults who are supposedly joined in a partnership of care. Coercive language appears to be entirely integrated into maternity service discourse. Maria-Sofie was told with her second pregnancy that she '*would have to be* induced on day 10'. Following the birth of her first baby, she was informed that she and her baby 'wouldn't be *allowed* to leave the hospital if the baby hadn't fed twice for 20 minutes'. A very basic psychology comes into play when assertive adults are told what they can and cannot do without being offered any explanation. They resort to defiance:

> So I just asked them to shut the curtains and when they came back an hour and a half later, they said, 'Has he fed?' And I said, 'Yes, he's fed for 20 minutes', and again, an hour and a half later, I said the same thing, so that ticked the box. They hadn't seen him feed, but I was allowed to come home and I phoned my community midwife who I liked and she came and helped me with the breastfeeding.

There are other forms of communication which aim to control women by suggesting to them that their emotional response to pregnancy is either overstated, childish or of no significance to busy professionals engaged in the hard, daily grind of providing care. Lili's story shows how undermining women's pleasure in their pregnancy leads them to believe that they are not, after all, as special as they feel and that, as far as their carers are concerned, they are simply one of many, rather than unique individuals. Lili became pregnant shortly after her wedding, and asked her GP whether she would be safe to fly in the first months of pregnancy. This was one of several encounters that belittled the excitement she was feeling:

> I spoke to my GP about flying and this was the first time I realized that people didn't necessarily think about birth as I imagined that they would. His attitude was very much, 'Don't bother coming to see me now because you might have a miscarriage anyway. Come back in about 12 weeks and we'll get you an appointment to go to the local hospital'. And that was it.
>
> A few weeks later, I met the midwife for my booking appointment and she was quite hostile. And I said to her, 'What are my options for where I could have the baby?' And she said, 'There is no way you can have a home birth'. So I came home quite upset. No-one had said,

'Congratulations! You're having a baby!' They just got cross with me for asking questions.

Anyway, I carried on seeing the midwife until 20 weeks and I mentioned home birth again and she basically said, 'You can't have one; stop bothering me'.

The failure to acknowledge and indeed to participate in the mother's delight in her pregnancy, and subsequently to engage in any discussion about her desire to have a home birth resulted in the mother losing confidence not only in the maternity service but also in herself. Respectful communication fosters the dignity of all those engaged in it, and increases the quality of professional and personal life. It is hard to imagine what possible benefit might be thought to accrue from attacking the mother's happiness, unless it increased the sense of importance of those conveying the message that, for them, the business of pregnancy was no more than a job they had to do.

Lili described how her encounters with her GP and midwife made her feel during the first half of her pregnancy:

In those first 20 weeks, I felt so upset about everything and I felt like I was always in trouble for something. I thought I don't really want this, I want to opt out.

She opted out by choosing to employ an independent midwife. Further encounters with staff merely served to confirm that she had made the right decision. Her pregnancy was prolonged and she went for a scan at 42 weeks:

The woman who did the scan said to me, 'This is ridiculous; your baby could die because you are not allowing yourself to be induced'. And the midwives' attitude was 'You are taking such a risk; I can't believe you are being so stupid'. And I did get slightly wobbly, thinking perhaps I was doing something really silly. But they also made me think, 'I don't want to be in your system; I'm fine on my own'.

Discussing abuse in hospital-based settings, Hodges (2009) describes how mothers' self-esteem can be undermined by 'threatening, scolding, ridiculing, shaming, mocking, dismissing and refusing to acknowledge' (p. 9), all of which were experienced by the women in this book. She discusses how women accept this kind of communication because they are socialized into expecting that health professionals will behave in a professional manner and therefore do not recognize behaviour which is definitely not professional.

The language and the tone of communication used by some of the health professionals whom the women encountered made them feel insecure and incompetent. It has been proposed that 'the 'real world' is to a large extent unconsciously built upon the language habits of the group' (Sapir 1958), that is, language creates the reality we experience. This is a major problem for midwifery; indeed, it is perhaps *the* major problem confronting the maternity service today. The language used in maternity care is creating, on a daily basis, a reality that is inimical to the ethos of midwifery, to midwives and to childbearing women. This language creates distrust in women in their own ability to carry a baby and give birth, and demeans the status of midwifery skills in the eyes of midwives by suggesting that skills beyond their remit are likely to be needed to ensure a safe pregnancy and labour. It creates fears about the risk of childbirth that are out of proportion to the actual risk of having a baby in the developed world in the twenty-first century. Language that induces fear appears to be the default position in maternity care; when events occur which prove that there was no need to be frightened, the embarrassment of having misread the situation is felt, not by the people who created the fear, but by the woman. Mia tells the story of her friend:

> A friend was told by the doctor that she had to go into the hospital for high blood pressure. She didn't have all the signs of pre-eclampsia, but she was told to go in. She was monitored for three days in the hospital and she was being told that her situation was life-threatening and that she was seriously ill and that she had to be induced, and that it would be completely foolish to delay the induction. They tried to break her waters; in fact, several people tried and then a doctor came to see her, looked at her notes, and said, 'Go home, I am not worried about you; come back when you are in labour'. So she came home but she said she felt ashamed leaving the hospital; she wanted to cover herself with her coat in case anybody saw her.

Margret spoke for many of the women in this book when she described the 'fear and apprehension' that she had felt as a result of being subjected to constant talk of risk. Even outcomes which had no risk implications were conveyed as being dangerous. Erin described how when her pregnancy had reached 41 weeks + 6 days, the Supervisor of Midwives asked to speak to her:

> She said, 'Our policy is to induce at 10 days over term'. And then she proceeded to tell me all the things that happen to babies that have very long pregnancies, *right down to the fact that they might have flaky skin*.

In a climate of risk-hysteria, even a perfectly normal phenomenon, such as flaky skin, is sucked into the risk vortex. When the maternity service talks constantly about what can go wrong, everybody – women, midwives and managers alike – ends up believing that risk is more prevalent than normality and that safety in childbirth is difficult to achieve. Women themselves are complicit in the creation of this new reality. Just as children acquire the turns of phrase and the favourite words used by their parents, so women who have not yet had babies acquire the language that they hear being used by other women when they tell their birth stories to each other. If that language is the language of fear, submission, intervention and helplessness, the next generation of women will expect and probably, therefore, experience that kind of childbirth reality. Staton-Savage (2001) describes how birth stories are a key component of informal communication of knowledge about childbirth to expectant mothers. She expresses concern that because the majority of births now take place in hospital, women's accounts of their labours are set within a medical context and conveyed through medical terminology. The woman's role in her labour is diminished and that of health professional staff is portrayed as central, so that the inheritance of today's childbearing women is 'a toxic legacy of attitudes about childbirth' (Arms, cited in Staton Savage 2001: 5). The absence of positive, woman-centred birth stories and their replacement with stories that put interventions in labour centre-stage mean that:

> An aberrant childbirth mythology evolves and may be passed from one generation to the next.
>
> (p. 5)

Language, however, can also be a tool for changing the system as well as reinforcing it. Prior to her second labour, Mette wrote a letter to her midwives which included a detailed birth plan. In it, she refers several times to what she has learned about the power of language to affect the course of labour, and suggests a different kind of language to enable her to birth more easily:

> I ask you more than anything to encourage me to *relax* into the *sensations* or *surges* (you might call them contractions) . . . I intend to *breathe through* the sensations and when it comes to crowning and my body *releasing* the baby, I ask you or my husband not to tell me to push, but instead (if I need it) to *breathe the baby out*. I do not want to be told it is all taking too long (given the length of my last birth, this is unlikely to be the case). I would like to experience the birth process without trauma or hurry.[Author's emphasis]

She highlights what she sees as the crucial importance of the language used during labour and birth by putting a box around her final request:

Please be very careful what you say in my presence about how I or the birth are doing.

In order to avoid the language of risk creating inaccurate perceptions of childbirth that lead to defensive practice on the part of health professionals and fear on the part of women, it is important to consider how risk can be presented accurately. At present, pregnant women are shown themselves in a mirror that distorts their true image as women competent emotionally and physically to birth their babies. The presentation of risk has exercised both business and health care for some time. John Palin has devised visual means of presenting risk which generate a discourse that creates a more accurate 'risk reality' than that which the everyday language of health care is tending to create at present. The Palin Palette© depicts 1000 stick figures on a single sheet of paper. If the risk of shoulder dystocia is 10 in 1000, ten of the stick figures are highlighted. The mother can then 'see' what her risk is and process it visually rather than through the medium of language. Ways such as these of reframing risk in health and maternity care are urgently required.

The language and mode of communication experienced by the women in this book tended to destroy the possibility of a relationship developing between woman and midwife, which would enable them both to feel empowered. Hunter *et al.* (2008) describe relationships as 'the hidden threads in the tapestry of maternity care' (p. 132) and suggest that low morale among midwives in the UK and other European countries may be due to working within a system that hinders relationship formation (p. 134). For the relationships to change, the language upon which their development depends has to change. If the only language women hear midwives using is that of risk, the fear created in them will lead to dependency on the people whom they perceive as able not only to define the risk but also to resolve it. A relationship of dependency is not what midwifery wants. An approach that fits its philosophy and objectives far more appropriately is one based on salutogenesis (Antonovsky 1987), a theory which proposes that it is better to identify and utilize people's own resources to manage their health than to make them dependent on resources outside themselves. Salutogenesis rejects the traditional focus on illness and incapacity within health services and aims to help people to understand themselves and their 'condition' better and therefore to move in a direction that will promote or, in the case of pregnant women, maintain health (as most pregnant women are not ill).

Proponents of salutogenesis focus on people's capacity to get well or stay well rather than adopting a pathological perspective which focuses on obstacles to their health and deficits in their personalities or lifestyles. It is a profoundly 'green' theory because it encourages people to find and use their own strengths, rather than creating dependency on extremely expensive and often wasteful technologies.

The women in this book manifested a strong inclination towards salutogenesis. They had a pervasive, enduring though dynamic feeling of confidence that:

(1)   the stimuli from one's internal and external environments in the course of living are structured, predictable and explicable;

(2)   the resources are available to meet the demands posed by these stimuli; and

(3)   these demands are challenges, worthy of investment and engagement.

(Antonovsky 1987: 19)

That is, they were confident that pregnancy and birth have an inherent anatomical and physiological logic as demonstrated by the proliferation of the human race down the centuries; they felt that they had the physical and psychological strength to give birth to their babies, and they welcomed the challenge of finding an environment that would make the experience of birthing one which would enhance their self-esteem and provide a positive foundation for motherhood.

Practice-based salutogenesis should be far more central to midwifery than it appears to many women currently to be. Downe and McCourt (2004) comment that it 'opens the door to turning the concept of risk systems on its head' (p. 18). It is a tool for promoting mental as well as physical health, because it focuses on helping people to make sense of the experiences they are having, and then to take control of the direction in which they are travelling. At a time when the incidence of mental illness associated with childbirth appears to be increasing, as indicated by the level of tokophobia, postnatal depression and post-traumatic stress syndrome, it seems important to try to develop a language that will create a new and far more positive reality for midwives to practise in and childbearing women to birth in. While Downe and McCourt (2004) advocate salutogenesis as a philosophy that maximizes the sense of coherence of the birthing woman; it also has the power to create that sense of coherence in midwifery as well.

Key points

- Health care services need clients who will say what they want and how they can be helped to achieve their goals.
- If women encounter criticism, impatience and negative attitudes, they will, in turn, start to criticize and threaten in an attempt to regain control.
- Practice dependent on technology escalates the cost of health care and endangers patients in situations where technology is not available.
- The language used in maternity care is creating a reality that is inimical to the ethos of midwifery and to childbearing women.

References

Antonovsky A. (1987) *Unravelling the Mystery of Health: How people manage stress and stay well*. San Francisco: Jossey-Bass.

Christensen H. and Mackinnon A. (2010) Cognition in pregnancy and motherhood: prospective cohort study. *The British Journal of Psychiatry* 196:126–32.

Department of National Health and Welfare Canada (1970) *The Canadian Mother and Child* (3rd ed.). Ottawa: Department of National Health and Welfare Canada.

Dimond B. (2005) Mental capacity and midwifery practice. *British Journal of Midwifery*, 13(4):233.

Downe S. and McCourt C. (2004) From being to becoming: reconstructing childbirth knowledges. In Downe S. (ed.) *Normal Childbirth: Evidence and debate*. Edinburgh: Churchill Livingstone: 3–24.

Frith L. and Draper H. (2004) *Ethics and Midwifery: Issues in contemporary practice*. London: Elsevier Books for Midwives.

Goodrich, F. H. (1967) *Preparing for Childbirth: A Manual for Expectant Parents*. London: George Allen and Unwin Ltd.

Hodges S. (2009) Abuse in hospital-based birth settings? *The Journal of Perinatal Education*, 18(4):8–11.

Hunter B., Berg M., Lundgren I., Olafsdottir A. and Kirkham M. (2008) Relationships: the hidden threads in the tapestry of maternity care. *Midwifery*, 24:132–7.

Jarrett C. (2010) The maternal brain. *The Psychologist*, 23(3):186–188.

Royal College of Midwives (2002) *Home Birth: Position Paper 25*. London: RCM.

Sapir E. (1958) *Culture, Language and Personality* (ed. D. G. Mandelbaum). Berkeley, CA: University of California Press.

Stapleton H., Kirkham M., Curtis P. and Thomas G. (2002) Silence and time in ante-natal care. *British Journal of Midwifery*, 10(6):393–6.

Staton Savage J. (2001) Birth stories: a way of knowing in childbirth education. *Journal of Perinatal Education*, 10(2):3–7.

Website

NHS leaflet for expectant fathers: tinyurl.com/lnl7ag (accessed 28 March 2010).

6 Avoidance, subversion and confrontation

In 2005, in Birmingham, Ruth Weston, an 'ordinary' mother, gave a speech at a midwifery conference during which she described her struggle to have the home water births she wanted for her babies. She explored her experiences through her understanding of liberation theology as she had tried to live it for many years as a church worker. Listening to her speech was the kind of experience which does not happen very often in a lifetime; Ruth Weston held the attention of the audience for every second that she was speaking – midwives, managers, academics and mothers alike. The audience instantly and unanimously recognized that what she was saying was right, that the analysis she was providing as a woman and mother of four children, rather than as a health professional, was cutting to the heart of what was wrong with the maternity service. It was a case where any resistance by professionals to 'being told how things should be' by a lay person melted away in the face of Ruth's passion and intelligence. The excuses and the prevarications which everyone present knew they had engaged in at some point while being a part of the maternity service, either as employee or as client, were laid bare and by the end of the speech, everyone was convinced that change was essential if the relationship between medicine, midwifery and women was not to become toxic and destructive of the integrity of all concerned. Ruth did not speak for very long but when she had finished, the audience did not merely rise to their feet, but leapt up to give her a standing, cheering ovation which it was difficult to quell. Many people were in tears. The conference was arrested for an indeterminate time until people regained control of their emotions.

> *Ruth described how* women have stopped believing in their bodies; they can no longer read its messages, and midwives are trained to defer to doctors and machines rather than their own eyes and hands and expertise of normal birth. *She felt that* the historical dominance of the male doctor and the medicalization of birth has produced a false dichotomy between the welfare of the mother and of the baby, pitting the welfare of the one against that of the other.

The stories of the women in this book illustrate very clearly the themes of

Ruth's speech, suggesting that her analysis is not limited to her own experiences, but has a far wider resonance. Perhaps the argument most commonly used to deter women from home birth, and especially if they want a home birth against medical advice, is that they will be putting the survival of their baby at risk. Yet common sense, drawing on a very basic understanding of the theory of evolution, makes it hard to believe that women will choose to jeopardize their babies' safety. Human beings are committed to the survival of the species through their own and their offspring's survival. Pregnant women are doubtless subject to an innate drive to protect their unborn child and do everything they can to ensure his or her safe arrival in the world. Experience of being with and talking to women tells us that they constantly put their unborn babies' interests in front of their own; in twenty-first century, Western terms, this means giving up activities which they normally enjoy, depriving themselves of everyday treats such as a glass of lager or a piece of soft cheese and going to immense lengths to observe the hundreds of commandments which government, medical and other authorities lay upon them in pregnancy.

Some women continue to smoke during pregnancy – is this not a case of women putting themselves before their babies? I do not think it's quite as simple as that. Firstly, many women try to give up smoking once they find they are pregnant and a proportion are successful. Quite a few more try to cut down on the number of cigarettes they have each day. Some genuinely believe that smoking is desirable because it will make their babies smaller and therefore easier to birth – a curious but not irrational twist of the evolutionary imperative. Women who continue to smoke will almost certainly feel guilty, suggesting that for whatever reason it is they are continuing to smoke, their pleasure in cigarettes is much reduced. Some women smoke because it is their primary strategy for coping with the stresses in their lives; without cigarettes, their stress would be perhaps more damaging to their unborn babies' well-being than the effect of cigarettes. The pathological sequelae of pregnancy stress are considered at some length in the next chapter.

Turning to the women in this book – all of whom were accused of selfishness in choosing to have a home birth – is it reasonable to suppose that a woman such as Erin whose first baby had died of a rare genetic condition and who had subsequently had a miscarriage would be likely to do anything that might put her third baby at risk? She had waited a long time to achieve a successful pregnancy. Her state of mind for the first two trimesters was one of continual anxiety for the baby's safety:

> With all of that behind me, I didn't really know when I got pregnant again what kind of birth I wanted. All I could think about was getting past 10 weeks when I had the miscarriage and then getting past 28 weeks because that's when I had the first baby. After that, it was like a new realm of possibility and I just thought, 'I might actually have a baby at the end of this'.

The women whose stories are told here did not differentiate between their own welfare and that of their babies; they did indeed feel that the maternity service was creating *a false dichotomy between the welfare of the mother and of the baby*. They believed that labour and birth were equally important to both parties and that both needed to be protected from harms which the mother could foresee and should therefore take steps to avoid. The women were not naïve; they knew that some of the harms which might threaten the welfare of mother and baby were iatrogenic and that the hospital environment created pressures for health care staff which affected their behaviour but which were unrelated to safeguarding mothers and babies. Mette describes an experience of hospital pressure of time forcing a decision that she was not ready to make:

> I said, 'Can I have five minutes to think about it?' [accepting a blood transfusion] and they said, 'Well, actually, we've got a lot of people we need to look after, so no, you can't, basically'. They put this emotional pressure on you to go along with what they think is best for you, but also what's the convenient thing for them to do quickly.

The women also noticed that arguments favouring medical intervention over nature's own processes did not always seem to have logic on their side. Alessia questioned her hospital's policy of inducing twins at 38 weeks:

> There's this obsession with making sure twin babies are born early. I put on half a stone in the last four weeks of pregnancy, not eating any differently. If the twins had been delivered at 38 weeks, they wouldn't have come out at the weight they did. They would have been underweight and they would have been put straight into a plastic box with monitors attached. I would have been unable to breastfeed. People say to me, 'They are good weights' and I say, 'Yes, there's a reason for that; they were born at term'. The reason twins are underweight is because they whip them out early; they're not ready. I mean, nature's very, very good at doing the job.

A study (Boucher *et al.* 2009) of the 1 per cent of women in the United States who choose home birth found that of 160 respondents, more than half possessed a college degree and many also held advanced degrees, suggesting that it is not through any lack of intelligence that women opt for home securities rather than the advanced obstetric technologies available in American hospitals. The researchers found that many of the women were motivated in their choice of home by a desire to have control over their birthing experience (p. 122).

The urge to control appears to be significant in many encounters between assertive women and professionals in maternity care. It was at the heart of nearly all the engagements the women in this book had with staff. Even after the safe arrival of Mette's baby, an attempt was made to 'control' her happiness and enforce retrospective acceptance that what the hospital had said about its being safer to give birth in a medical environment was right, and that she was simply lucky not to have had any problems:

> The midwife said to me, 'Well, just because you play chicken and egg on a motorway and don't get run over doesn't mean you did the right thing!'

From the women's point of view, the control that others were trying to have over them at this most important juncture of their lives was oppression. In her speech in Birmingham, Ruth Weston (2005) spoke of how to combat oppression and described three strategies of *avoidance, subversion* and *confrontation*. All of these were employed by the women in this book. If the maternity service is truly trying to listen to women and to enable as many as possible to participate on an equal footing in their own care with health professionals, there are some interesting insights to be gained from exploring both why and how some women deliberately avoid engaging with it.

The NHS is committed to increasing access to its services. A recent document on the maternity service is subtitled, 'Choice, *access* and continuity of care in a safe service' (DH 2007) and states in the 'executive summary' that the government's aim is to provide 'high quality, safe and *accessible* services that are both women-focused and family-centred' (p. 5). Yet according to Weston (2005), avoidance is practiced by both mothers and midwives:

> It is where you circumvent or bypass the system altogether. So you become an independent midwife or you engage an independent midwife, or go to a birthing centre or plan an unassisted birth.

Avoidance was the principal strategy that the women in this book used to retain control over their bodies, their births and their babies. Margret, Alessia, Lea, Lili, Maria-Sofie and Leonie decided that the most effective way to escape the maternity service's drive to control was to employ an independent midwife, even though this was difficult for all of them to afford. Lea explained that having an independent midwife *took all the pressure off*, liberating her to start enjoying her pregnancy. Lili, a firm believer in the principles of the NHS, was hesitant about contacting an independent midwife. However, the midwife's positive response to her situation was so refreshing that the question of finding her fee immediately became a problem that could be managed:

> I said, 'What do you think – is home birth on an island ridiculous?' And she said, 'Well, no, it's not an issue. If you want me to come and meet you, I will'. She came over and she was so amazingly positive. We decided that even if it meant borrowing, begging or stealing the money, we would get hold of it.

For Alessia, meeting two independent midwives who were prepared to help her have her twins at home was:

> . . . like knights in shining armour coming to our rescue; it was just the most amazing feeling that somebody out there was willing to come and help us.

The women's relief at finally being free of the maternity service was almost certainly the same desire for freedom that had driven the independent midwives who attended their births to work outside the system. The current threat to independent midwifery could be seen as another manifestation of the health service's drive to enforce conformity on practitioners and consumers alike. Conformity and choice are very uneasy bed-fellows, and attacking independent midwives does not add credence to the government's rhetoric of choice.

Independent midwives can be seen as the guardians of midwifery precisely because they have to develop and maintain a wide range of *midwifery* skills in order to work in the woman's home without the availability of drugs and technology. Their skills have to be fine-tuned because their practice appears to be subjected to much closer scrutiny than that of colleagues working in hospital settings. Beverley Beech (2009: 4) notes that a disproportionate number of independent midwives are reported to the Nursing and Midwifery Council (NMC), and speculates whether this is a concerted effort to remove them from the register. She considers that double standards are in operation so that when women complain about care received in hospital, internal enquiries are set in motion; but when complaints are made against community or independent midwives, it is far more likely that the midwife will be referred to the NMC. Margret's midwife considered Margret's pregnancy to be the 'most normal' that she'd undertaken for a long time, but when she spoke to her Supervisor of Midwives, she was warned:

> 'You've got to tread carefully with this birth because of the action plan the Trust's put in. If anything does go wrong, they're going to be after your pin number'.

Given the fact that independent midwives have only their own skills to rely on when they are with a woman at a home birth, and given the rigorous surveillance to which they are subjected, it seems an eminently rational decision to choose to employ one when maternity service midwives are saying that they do not have the skills to assist women with complex pregnancies to give birth to their babies. The response given to Alessia's request for a home birth was:

> . . . that the midwives weren't competent, they weren't confident and they certainly weren't trained to deal with this,

leading Alessia to speculate on when in the last 50 years midwives had lost their skills to help a woman give birth to twins at home.

Margret did not consider an independent midwife until the very end of her pregnancy. By this point, she was so desperate to find the support she needed to help her achieve both the physical and emotional sense of safety that she craved, that she was driven to consider free birthing in order to avoid the maternity service:

> I had a discussion with my husband about it. I said, 'It's my fourth baby; how would you feel if we just didn't ring them?' And he said, 'Well, if it's what you want to do, I'll trust your judgement. We could ring them right at the very end, depending on how you're feeling, how things are going'.

Simply not to call the midwives was the ultimate expression of avoidance and as far as Margret and her husband were concerned, very much a last resort. For a small minority of women, it is the first resort when they realize that the maternity service is not going to offer them what they feel is essential for them to have an 'ecological birth' – one which uses no resources but the internal resources of the mother and her supporters, and which results in no harm being done at any level – physical, psychological or spiritual – to anyone present at the birth. The story of one such woman is told in chapter 8 and is the most extreme form of avoidance, as discussed by Ruth Weston.

Weston (2005) notes that avoidance is a costly strategy for those who employ it. Midwives who avoid working in the maternity service by choosing to practise outside it give up financial and legal security, and subject themselves to relentless scrutiny, apparently designed to catch them out. Women who engage independent midwives pay a large fee which, at the point of starting or expanding their family, is often difficult to find. Weston describes avoidance as 'a difficult road' but as an important step because it forces the maternity service to look at why some women find avoidance necessary and may result in elements of the care that the women are forced to seek outside the service being incorporated into it. Weston (2005) claims that avoidance shows that alternatives to the statutory service are *realistic, workable* and *effective*.

The second strategy which Weston (2005) discussed in her conference speech is *subversion*, which she described as 'the valid defence of the powerless'. Subversion can be very creative, as Margret demonstrated when she refused to have any scans so that her midwives and doctors would not know how large her baby was:

> We went along until 38 weeks with the midwives every now and again hinting at the fact that this baby was huge, but I didn't have any scans because I didn't want there to be any evidence that they could beat me with. I wanted not to give them any ammunition really.

Mia behaved subversively in order to find out what had been the reason for the caesarean that she had undergone with her first baby. To do this, she needed to obtain her medical records, but because she was poor and because, in any case, she objected to having to pay to see her own notes, she arranged for a friend who worked in Medical Records to obtain them for her so that she could read them overnight. In them she found a letter which had been written by the consultant at the hospital where her baby had been born to the consultant at her present hospital. The note read:

> Don't know why she had a c section with her first. Could have been CPD [cephalo-pelvic disproportion]; or maybe everybody just got bored.

Obtaining her records in this way was probably legally questionable. Mia, however, felt that it was her right to have information that was crucial to her decision-making in her current pregnancy. The lack of a medical reason for the caesarean made her very angry and also justified in her own eyes the subversive action she had taken to obtain her notes. The way in which her first child had been born had been one of the determining factors in leading her to have her second baby in hospital and had continued to cause difficulties for her when she requested a home birth for her third baby.

All of the women subverted the system by joining groups where what Freire (1972) describes as the 'culture of domination' was challenged, and where they found support. Home birth groups were used by the women to gain ideas on how to get what they wanted and provided a locus of opposition where dissenters could find the strength to continue to resist the pressures placed on them to conform. Mia noted that:

> The Home Birth Support Group was only contacted by people who needed extra support. I have met women who wanted home births and they got support for it, so they never contacted the Group. It's the others. By its very title really, it's going to be selective for women who haven't got the medical support.

She met 'amazing women' at the group who had not had a medical blessing for their home births, and who helped her to understand what kind of birth she wanted:

> It's astounding how powerful it is and the difference it made. There are women all around the place who have been truly empowered by it. And it cast light on what happened the first time for me and made me think, 'hang on – they told me it had to be like that; how come they never told me it could be like this?!'

Maria-Sofie spoke of the importance of belonging to a Home Birth Group where she:

... learned a lot from the other women locally who have also had to fight the maternity care system and the policies in R . . .

The third of the strategies for challenging oppression is *confrontation*, considered by Weston (2005) to be the most difficult of the three, which women may use to achieve their freedom:

> This is the difficult one because we are so well conditioned not to make a fuss and do as we are told. And if we are nice, nobody listens, but if we get angry we are dismissed as emotional neurotic bitter women . . . Sadly the feminism of the last century has not overturned these cultural norms particularly in the maternity services.

Most of the women simply avoided the system or quietly subverted it. A couple, however, confronted it head on to demonstrate either the illogicality of its position or the dishonesty of its processes. Alessia's run-in with her maternity service made headline news in the local press, publicity which she had not sought but which she was nonetheless prepared to use to advance her case. In her meetings with health staff, she exposed on more than one occasion the deceits which she considered had been practised upon her. At the third meeting with the Head of Midwives and the Supervisor of Midwives to discuss her home birth, when she was 36 weeks pregnant, Alessia was informed that the Trust's legal team had been consulted and was advising that the Trust did not offer home birth. Alessia immediately highlighted the deviousness of waiting to give her this information until she was so late in her pregnancy that either continuing to fight or make alternative arrangements for the birth of her babies would be difficult:

> Well, what the hell have we been talking about then for the last three meetings?

The Head of Midwives justified the Trust's position by explaining that 'her midwives' were not allowed to act outside their remit and 'do things that they are not trained to do, such as attending water births or the birth of twins at home'. Alessia countered with the argument that 'her midwives' were clearly in need of further training. Following this meeting, Alessia sought the help of Beverley Beech at the Association for Improvements in the Maternity Services (AIMS), an organization very well known for its willingness to confront medical and midwifery hierarchies when it perceives that women are being oppressed. She also went online to a midwives' yahoo group, made her situation public and asked for help. As a result of this direct action, she finally got the support of three independent midwives who agreed to help her without charging their usual fee which she and her husband could not afford.

Alessia couched her analysis of what had happened to her very much in political terms. She saw her treatment by the maternity service as an attack on values she held dearly. Profoundly challenged in her trust in democracy, she explained the contradictions which she felt she had detected:

> We live in a country where we are allowed freedom of speech and freedom of choice and in practice, this is definitely not the case. But we're told every day that it is. So I felt totally cheated.

Leaving aside the question of whether allowing people to participate in their own care to the point where they have complete control over their health choices, it is interesting to look further afield and set the NHS rhetoric of choice and participation in the context of human rights. Article 8 of the Human Rights Act (1998) concerns the '[r]ight to respect for private and family life'. This is elaborated in the International Covenant on Economic, Social and Cultural Rights (1976) which provides in Article 10 for:

> The widest possible protection and assistance . . . to the family, which is the natural and fundamental unit of society, *particularly for its establishment* and while it is responsible for the care and education of dependent children. [Author's emphasis]

It might be contested that the right to respect for family life was, in fact, violated by the treatment the women in this book received as a result of their choice to give birth to their babies in the place which would become the baby's home. Women who favour home birth often talk about birth as a domestic event, which should take place where the family lives. Similarly, many people would prefer to die at home, because death is part of the continuum of family life and should be experienced within the context of that life. The women fought to create their family in the way that seemed most protective of family values. Attempts to control and distort their family life by insisting that they give birth in hospital were viewed by them as an attack on a basic need and a fundamental right.

   Article 8 of the Human Rights Act continues by stating that a public authority (such as the maternity service) cannot interfere with the right to respect for family life except under certain conditions, one of which is 'for the protection of health' and another 'for the protection of the rights and freedoms of others'. Whether, were such a case ever to come to court, the protection of the health, rights and freedoms of the unborn baby might be considered to outweigh the mother's right to family life by giving birth at home would provide the material for an interesting legal debate. Once again, we would be looking at the erroneous dichotomy between the welfare of the mother and the baby, and the implication that the welfare of the baby should over-ride the mother's right to have control over her own body. An incident which focused this issue in the popular mind took place in 2009 and made headline news in both the tabloid and broadsheet press:

A pregnant woman was refused a drink at a pub and then asked to leave by staff who said they were protecting her unborn child. Caroline Williams, 26, who is five months pregnant, says she felt humiliated by the treatment. She insists she is a responsible mother and would never endanger her baby . . . She said: 'I was on a rare night out with some friends. I had a pint of lager and a friend offered to get me another half – that was going to be my limit. He was refused service because it was for me and when I later took a sip from another friend's glass, the assistant manageress asked me and my friends to leave'.

(Daily Mail 2009)

A Professor of Psychology (Gross 2010) commenting on the affair, construed it as yet another indication of the intrusion of public concern, not necessarily well-informed, into the pregnant mother's space and a reflection on a culture which views pregnant women as not best placed to understand their baby's needs. Is there a difference between intervening when an adult is hitting a child and intervening when a pregnant woman smokes a cigarette or drinks a pint of lager? Should the responsible citizen see both as occasions when his or her conscience requires action? Does the woman 'own' her unborn child or does society/the health service/the legal system? These are issues that we need to be clear about because they go to the heart of the debate about choice in maternity care.

Stapleton *et al.* (2002) noted in their informed choice study that most women expected to conform with the kind of care that the maternity service routinely provides. Women who had concerns and who wanted to discuss them were labelled as trouble-makers and tended to attract a hostile reception from the professionals with whom they came into contact. There was, for most women, no sense of being on an equal footing with their caregivers and this made raising objections to what was being suggested difficult and generally impossible.

In order to make choices, a woman has to be free to do so, and that means being free to apply information to her personal circumstances and reach her own conclusions without fear that the quality of her care might be affected if she makes the 'wrong' choice. Given that there is genuine freedom to make a choice, she must then assume responsibility for whatever is the outcome of her choice (provided that health staff have practised to the standards expected of their profession). Many of us find taking responsibility for our health care daunting, and choose, by not making choices, to place the responsibility for outcomes on health professionals' shoulders.

The issue of responsibility around health and health care is one of the major challenges for citizens of the twenty-first century. Failing to take responsibility for personal health has led to escalating levels of chronic disease in rich populations – the diseases associated with undisciplined lifestyles – poor diet, smoking, lack of exercise, alcohol abuse. Yet the fault does not lie entirely with the general public. For years, medicine has implied that it can both diagnose and treat any illness or state of dis-ease. People have presumed that there is an easy fix for whatever harm they inflict on their bodies. We are now increasingly and uncomfortably aware that medicine does not have the answer to all our problems and that, even if it did, the country cannot afford to make all possible treatments available to everyone. As the public becomes more aware that there are limits to what the health service can provide, and that the evidence to which health professionals refer is never quite as robust as they might hope, making choices about what kind of health care one wants may become less attractive than making an effort to stay healthy and avoid having to make those choices in the first place.

Choice in maternity care remains very challenging to women who have for years had the responsibility of labour and birth taken away from then. Following the Peel Report of 1970 (DHSS), all women were strongly encouraged to have their babies in hospital. This had multiple consequences; the rate of home birth dropped to an all-time low, extinguishing both the confidence and many of the traditional skills of the midwife, and women naturally assumed that, having taken the advice to come into hospital, whatever happened while they were there was someone else's responsibility. Tragedies occurred, babies and sometimes mothers died, but there was always someone to blame. Obstetrics and midwifery have created the circumstances under which litigation around childbirth has become the most burdensome in all of medicine. When women choose, however, to have their babies at home, they accept that they are out of immediate reach of technology and certain professional expertise, and that at least some of the responsibility for what happens rests with them. This would seem a win-win situation for both women and health professionals and also for the government agenda to develop a more mature understanding and experience of partnership in health care.

Freedom is inseparable from responsibility. One way of avoiding responsibility is to conform. Making no choices by allowing an institution, through its policies and protocols, to make them for us is one way of conforming. Of course, we may agree with the policies and protocols and therefore believe that the institution can safely be left to make choices on behalf of health care consumers. Such a position, however, depends on firstly knowing what the policies and protocols are and secondly, having thought them through critically. Only under these circumstances can we make a genuine choice to give our allegiance rather than merely giving it blindly.

The women in this book took their choices very seriously, but also accepted responsibility for the outcomes of their choices. While challenge is painful for both mothers and professionals, to comply with care which does not enable one to realize personal values is to deny one's right to a full humanity. Freire (1972) would describe this as being fearful of freedom. Freedom brings with it autonomy and responsibility, qualities which a mature health service must learn to recognize and value in both its clients and its workforce. The women in this book went through considerable emotional turmoil to achieve what they felt was their right. It is interesting that Freire described liberation as 'a childbirth and a painful one'.

Key points

- The maternity service is creating a false dichotomy between the welfare of the mother and of the baby. They are inter-dependent.
- The urge to control is prominent in encounters between women and professionals.
- Women will avoid care in order to retain control over their bodies, their births and their babies.
- In the UK today, it appears that pregnant women are not considered best placed to understand their baby's needs.
- Freedom brings with it autonomy and responsibility, qualities which a mature health service recognizes and values in both its clients and its workforce.

References

Beech B. (2009) Midwifery: running down the drain. *AIMS Journal*, 21(3):3–5.

Boucher D., Bennett C., McFarlin B. and Freeze R. (2009) Staying home to give birth: why women in the United States choose home birth. *Journal of Midwifery and Women's Health*, 54:1109–126.

Department of Health (2007) *Maternity matters: choice, access and continuity of care in a safe service*. London: DH.

Department of Health and Social Security (1970) Standing Maternity and Midwifery Advisory Committee (J. Peel, Chairman) *Domiciliary Midwifery and Maternity Bed Needs*. London: HMSO.

Freire P. (1972) *Pedagogy of the Oppressed*. Harmondsworth: Penguin Books.

Gross H. (2010) Taking up space: pregnancy in public. *The Psychologist*, 23(3):202–4.

Stapleton H., Kirkham M., Curtis P. and Thomas G. (2002) Silence and time in ante-natal care. *British Journal of Midwifery*, 10(6):393–6.

Weston R. Sharples (2005) Liberating childbirth. *AIMS Journal*, 17(3), available online at www.aims.org.uk/Journal/Vol17No3/liberatingChildbirth.htm (accessed 2 April 2010).

Websites

Daily Mail 31 March 2009, 'Mother-to-be is ordered out of pub by staff concerned for health of her baby': www.dailymail.co.uk/news/article-1166124/Mother-ordered-pub-staff-concerned-health-baby.html#ixzz0jTvON6Tf (accessed 28 March 2010).

Human Rights Act: www.opsi.gov.uk/acts/acts1998/ukpga_19980042_en_3 (accessed 28 March 2010).

International Convenant on Economic, Social and Cultural Rights: www2.ohchr.org/english/law/cescr.htm (accessed 28 March 2010).

Ruth Weston: Liberating childbirth: www.aims.org.uk/Journal/Vol17No3/liberating Childbirth.htm (accessed 2 April 2010).

7   Stress in pregnancy and birth

All of the women in this book had stressful pregnancies. However confident they were in their decisions and however strong the support they received from their partners, independent midwives and home birth groups, there remained anxiety that affected the quality of their lives. Some described near pathological anxiety arising from simply being pregnant because it rekindled the memory of a traumatic first birth:

> My first was a caesarean birth and it was one of the worst days of my life. And then about a year later, I was pregnant again and I felt very anxious and I really didn't know what to do about my anxiety. I phoned the midwife and I think I must have used certain key words that they respond to because my named midwife came to see me and she was using the word 'anxious'.
>
> Mia

Mette thought that she had recovered from the physical and emotional problems caused by the severe tear she suffered when her first child was born. However, it became very apparent to her when she went to an antenatal appointment during her second pregnancy and was asked to give a sample of blood, that she was still profoundly affected by what had happened. She could not go through with the procedure:

> After that, I realized that I was traumatized. I thought I had got over the birth very positively, but there were definitely some underlying things going on that the visit to the clinic triggered. I was gutted for the rest of the day and really upset. I went away on a healing retreat at a Christian village and I just wanted to be healed from the trauma that had happened.

Erin had been through a first pregnancy in which she had discovered at 28 weeks that her baby had life-threatening problems. Following a week of sleeplessness, she and her partner decided on a termination:

For the sake of my mental health, I couldn't go on and try and complete the pregnancy, knowing that she could be stillborn at any time. So it was a really awful time.

This experience inevitably coloured her next two pregnancies, making her especially vulnerable to any suggestion that things might be going wrong. During her third pregnancy, she had to be constantly assertive in order to defend her decision to have a home birth. Her stress increased when she went overdue and started attending the hospital for twice-weekly scans:

> Every time I went in, the Supervisor of Midwives would wait for me outside the scan room and once I'd had all my monitoring, she would invite me to talk with her and on one occasion, she said, 'Our policy is to induce at 10 days over term' and she proceeded to tell me all the things that happen to babies that have very long pregnancies. It was really stressful and I wrote a letter and it basically said that if we were to experience the same thing again, then we would consider it harassment.

Once the women had gone over their due dates, health staff brought extra pressure to bear in order to persuade them to come into hospital to have their babies. The extra stress, in addition to what they had already experienced in relation to their decision to have a home birth, made this 'the most traumatic time' according to Lea.

Alessia was in conflict with the Head of Midwives from 25 weeks of pregnancy, a conflict which involved several rancorous meetings, an extensive and hostile correspondence with the hospital, publicity in the local press and the involvement of the Trust's legal team. Although she was buoyed up by anger at the way she was being treated, Alessia nonetheless described the last months of her pregnancy as 'horrible – you shouldn't as prospective parents have to go through such an ordeal'.

Margret describes her state of mind in the final weeks of her pregnancy and how she feared that the stress of insisting on a home birth would not be alleviated even when she went into labour:

> I did feel like I was being bullied, being pushed into a corner. I wasn't being given any option but to say, 'OK: I'll do it your way; I'll go into hospital'. I didn't want a hospital birth at home which was what they were offering, with troops of people in the house. I didn't want to have to battle when I was in labour.

Since Hans Selye (1982) first used the term *stress* in a biological context in the 1930s, an ever-increasing number of studies have demonstrated the adverse effects on the human immune system of prolonged or intense stress, leading to allergic responses, increased susceptibility to infection, gastro-intestinal problems, high blood pressure, stroke and heart attack. More recently, interest has focused on the effects of maternal stress during pregnancy on the unborn child. In 1993, Wadhwa *et al.* published a paper on the association between antenatal maternal stress, infant birth weight and gestational age at birth. This was a prospective study of 90 women who came from a similar socio-demographic background. The study controlled for each woman's level of biomedical risk and for her parity. In the third trimester, the women completed standardized questionnaires that measured different kinds of stress and pregnancy-related anxiety. The more stressed the women declared themselves to be, the more likely they were to give birth prematurely and to have a low birthweight baby. The researchers concluded that: 'Independent of biomedical risk, maternal prenatal stress factors are significantly associated with infant birth weight and with gestational age at birth' (p. 858).

O' Connor *et al.* (2002), in an article from the Avon Longitudinal Study of Parents and Children, reported on data collected from 7448 women who had completed several antenatal and postnatal assessments of anxiety and depression. The researchers wanted to test the hypothesis that antenatal maternal anxiety might predict behavioural problems in their children at four years of age. The evidence suggested that the pregnant woman's mood could have a direct effect on foetal brain development, with later consequences for the behavioural development of the child.

Studies have continued to be published that appear to demonstrate a link between the mother's stress levels during her pregnancy and both the physical and mental well-being of her child. In 2008, researchers from Harvard Medical School presented their findings on predisposition to asthma at the American Thoracic Society's International Conference in Toronto. They found that the level of stress experienced by the mother during pregnancy was related to how seriously her unborn child's immune system was affected by her exposure to dust. Even if the mother was exposed to low levels of dust at home during pregnancy, her child might be born highly allergic if the mother had also been very stressed. This study controlled for the mother's race, class, education and smoking history. The principal investigator commented that 'Stress can be thought of as a social pollutant that, when 'breathed' into the body, may influence the body's immune response similar to the effects of physical pollutants like allergens, thus adding to their effects' (www.sciencedaily.com).

In 2005, Austin *et al.* carried out a computerized review of the evidence from both published and unpublished animal studies about the impact of prenatal stress on the neural functioning and behaviour of offspring. The authors concluded that the findings from such studies might be applicable to humans and that more research into the role of maternal stress and anxiety during pregnancy was urgently required. In 2007, Egliston *et al.* agreed that the evidence from animal models was strong in suggesting that prenatal stress and anxiety experienced by the mother during sensitive periods of her unborn offspring's development could lead to permanent changes in its neurodevelopment and therefore behaviour.

Talge *et al.* (2007) reviewed evidence from independent prospective studies which found that if a mother is stressed while pregnant, her child is substantially more likely to have emotional and cognitive problems. This may be because there is a strong correlation between maternal and foetal cortisol levels. The authors concluded that the mechanisms involved in this interaction were only beginning to be understood.

Such a body of accumulating evidence must give us pause and oblige us to enquire whether the multiple stressors to which women are being subjected during pregnancy might be exacting a heavy price in terms of both the women's mental and physical health and their children's. This is likely to be a difficult and probably impossible equation to work out – how much stress is acceptable in physiological terms before a point is reached at which damage to the foetus might occur? How much pregnancy surveillance is safe before the mother's heightened sense of being 'at risk' leads to her and her baby actually being at risk? Is the relentless rota of antenatal visits and investigations to which pregnant women are subjected giving rise to long-term effects of which we have currently very little knowledge and which may be far more serious than anyone at the moment can grasp? Given the uncertain state of our understanding, might it not be best to play it safe and concentrate on protecting the emotional state of women (Odent 2004)?

In traditional societies, it is customary to make considerable efforts to protect the pregnant woman from stress. She becomes an almost sacred object with everyone in her community striving to safeguard her from both real and imagined harms. Pregnancy cravings are taken very seriously as indications of a physiological need. In other words, the pregnant woman is considered to be the expert on her own body and to have an intuitive and sound understanding of what she needs to ensure the healthy development of her baby. However, ancient cultures moved well beyond the physical in conceptualizing the relationship between the pregnant woman and her unborn child. The Chinese believed and believe that what affects a woman's mind will also affect the unborn baby in the womb. She is therefore encouraged to be calm and to surround herself with beautiful things during pregnancy. Before she goes to sleep at night, it is important for her to read or be told uplifting stories to ensure a positive frame of mind while she is dreaming. Chinese traditional practices during pregnancy also include singing; this is considered to be both physiologically and psychologically beneficial for the woman. Singing requires deep and steady breathing which helps the mother to relax and ensures a good oxygen supply to the baby inside her womb. In addition, singing promotes calm in both mother and unborn baby, a calm which will affect the child's temperament after birth. Michel Odent rediscovered this age-old custom when he initiated singing sessions for pregnant women at his clinic in Pithiviers.

The tradition of singing during pregnancy is also found in India where fine music was thought to be very favourable for the healthy development of unborn children. In Russia, at the beginning of the twentieth century, the importance of music was recognized at institutional level when the famous Russian obstetrician, Dmitry Ott, insisted that a concert hall should be built at his hospital, complete with organ. His pregnant patients were encouraged to attend the weekly musical events which were mounted there (www.english. pravda.ru). In Jewish mysticism, the Rabbis teach the importance of undertaking auspicious practices, known as 'segulot', during pregnancy to assist in the healthy development of the baby. This teaching moves perception of the special connection between mother and unborn baby from the physical and emotional levels, to the spiritual, so that the mother's spiritual state and the spiritual development of the foetus are also considered to be symbiotic (www.jewishpregnancy.org).

The sense of there being forces at play in the creation of a new human being that it may be difficult to articulate at the scientific level, but which are nonetheless very powerful, is deeply embedded in many ancient cultures and traditional societies. This is the kind of understanding of 'unknown unknowns', of acknowledging that human beings are subject to complex influences at all stages in their growth and development, that Hamlet famously expressed:

> There are more things in heaven and earth, Horatio,
> Than are dreamt of in your philosophy.
> (*Hamlet*, Act 1, Scene 5, lines 166–167)

An eminent professor of psychiatry once confided that he felt many of the problems which he saw in his Mother and Baby Unit had their origins in the way in which women were treated during their pregnancies and the interventions they were subjected to during labour. The modern-day equivalent of the rituals and practices which women in previous centuries followed is the schedule of clinic appointments, blood tests, scans and CTG monitoring, which structure the nine months of pregnancy today. The limitation of this approach to antenatal care is that it focuses exclusively on trying to detect physical problems in the mother and baby. It does not recognize the mother's psychological need to feel safe, or take into account the possible impact that maternal stress generated by repeated testing for pathologies during pregnancy might have on the biochemical status of the foetus. There is, of course, no acceptance in modern antenatal care that the foetus might in fact have a psychological and spiritual life which is developing concurrently with its organs and which might be equally susceptible to pregnancy 'insults'. As one midwife expressed at a recent international conference, maternity services do not recognize that, 'Prenatal care is what the mother does in between visits to the doctor and midwife' (Tritten 2010). It is the mother who is the principal carer of her unborn baby and it is what happens in her everyday life that most critically affects the health of her pregnancy. Even in law, there is recognition that mothers need 'protection' during pregnancy. The International Convenant on Economic, Social and Cultural Rights states that, 'Special protection should be accorded to mothers during a reasonable period before and after childbirth'.

Some professionals are beginning to write and speak about shifting the emphasis in antenatal care from the physical welfare of mother and baby to the emotional. Slade and Cree (2010) recommend that health professionals should:

> Provide specifically targeted emotional care for women from early in the pregnancy . . . This phase of life may be the most critical one of all for the new individual in that the baby's brain and central nervous system is developing. Having input to the well-being of women in pregnancy may be the most help we can ever be at an individual and societal level.
>
> (p. 194)

The women whose stories are told in this book were prepared to pay a heavy price in terms of the stress they experienced during pregnancy in order to achieve a relaxed labour at home. They did not believe that a hospital environment could provide them with the multi-faceted safety that they considered essential to labour effectively.

The lack of emotional security provided by health professionals during their pregnancies forced them to seek it elsewhere. They found it principally in the unstinting support of their partners (discussed at greater length in chapter 7) and also through attending Home Birth Support Groups. These groups provided the stability and the stress-free environment that Verny and Weintraub (2002) have described as having a significant impact on the healthy development of babies. They were the equivalent of Odent's piano sessions at Pithiviers. Odent notes (2007) that it is characteristic of the twenty-first century that women tend to be isolated at stages of their lives when they are especially in need of peer group contact, most notably during pregnancy and while breastfeeding. His clinic at Pithiviers was designed to provide strong social support which enabled the women to feel confident and happy as they waited to give birth to their babies and again in the early postnatal period. Many of the women in this book drew on the social support provided by home birth groups to enable them to feel positive about the choices they were making, and safe.

At the biochemical level, positive contact with others such as while hugging, sharing a meal or playing sport for fun, stimulates the release of oxytocin, a hormone which has an important relationship with sociability (Uvnäs-Moberg 2003). It plays a key part in sex, childbirth, mother/infant bonding, and breastfeeding, creating a feeling of relaxation and calm. It is antagonized by the stress hormone, adrenaline. During labour, while a certain amount of adrenaline will enable the woman to rise to the challenge of contractions, too much will cause her oxytocin levels to fall. As oxytocin is responsible for uterine contractions, the result of stress is that her labour slows down. This is probably an evolutionary mechanism to ensure that the woman does not give birth when she is in danger. Diminished oxytocin and heightened adrenaline create anxiety and diminish the pleasure that the mother feels in bringing her baby into the world. The women in this book who chose to have their babies at home were seeking an oxytocin-favourable environment which would enhance the emotional quality and physical progress of their labours.

Oxytocin flows most freely when the neocortex of the brain, which is stimulated by lights, noise and conversation, is quiescent. At an intuitive level, Erin was acutely aware of this as demonstrated by her behaviour in moving around the house to avoid distraction, and the planning she had done so as not to have to explain her wishes while actually in labour:

> Contractions started getting really powerful and I was using breathing techniques to get through each one. My partner started filling the pool. I went upstairs, didn't like it, and came straight back down but by then, the pool was full and I wasn't distracted from my breathing by the noise of the water and the practical things my partner was doing. So I got in the pool and it was about half seven in the morning; the sun was just coming up. The pool was in our living room. We had a tiny little house and we told the midwives to put their things in a different room and we put the birth plan on every door of the house so they didn't have to talk to me. Everything was perfect; it was just where I needed to be. I had privacy, the height of the water in the pool was perfect. I was warm. It was just ideal.

She felt a profound need for a peaceful atmosphere, and spoke of the disruption caused by a midwife who didn't initially sense what she was trying to achieve:

> The second midwife arrived a bit later and she had this rustly paper bag and she came up to me and said, 'What do you want to do about third stage?' right in the middle of a contraction. And at one point, she did get really loud and the other midwife told her to go into their room if she wanted to make a noise and after that, she got in line.

Leonie's account of her labour also focused on her need to concentrate on what was happening in her body, with nothing to distract her:

> The contractions began to take over. I found myself on all fours. They were coming upon me in waves and I had to hold on for dear life. The idea of pain relief had not crossed my mind. Very bizarre. I truly believe that any pain relief would have diverted me from the task at hand. I needed to be in total control of my faculties.

This need for quiet and privacy, which is so difficult to achieve in a delivery room in hospital or even within the more home-from-home environment of a midwife-led unit, was strongly expressed in the behaviour of the women during labour:

> I spent a lot of time in the pool on my own which was great because I knew there were people in the background, but I had my music on, I had some candles, it was all very dark and I felt fine throughout.
>
> Lili

Michel Odent (2010) has commented that the labouring woman needs to feel unobserved, but secure. There should be no-one closely around her, but only a mature, calm and silent midwife or doula in the background. Pascali-Bonaro and Kroeger (2004) have noted that the effect of encountering strangers during labour, even when they are committed to the care of the woman, creates fear and anxiety and enhances pain, leading them to conclude that a busy clinical environment with frequent changes of staff may not be conducive to effective labour. In a Cochrane Review of the evidence around continuous support during labour, Hodnett *et al.* (2007) also confirm that such support appears to be more effective when not provided by hospital staff.

The control Mia felt and the privacy she enjoyed, because for long periods the midwives stayed out of the room in which she was labouring, enabled her to concentrate so well on what was happening in her body that she was able to detect that her baby was not descending through her pelvis in the normal position. The undisturbed attention she was able to give to her labour enabled her to understand that this labour was different from her previous ones:

> Morning came and I started to feel some pressure to push, but it was not normal and I thought, 'I didn't think this baby was all that big, but this baby feels as wide as a bus'. I hadn't used any gas and air so I had nothing at all inhibiting my sensation and I felt skull in my pelvis. It felt grindingly difficult and different . . . And I pushed him out, and he was posterior and that's why it was so difficult. Nobody knew until he was born.

What these women describe is mammalian birth, rather than obstetric birth, and they managed to create the conditions which Tricia Anderson (2002) described when she advised midwives to reflect on what cats need to give birth and the consequences of disturbing their labour by the presence of people, bright lights and noise. Disruptions in labour may be treated in the delivery suite by syntocinon augmentation followed by epidural to help the mother cope with the increased intensity of her contractions. Both interventions lead to disturbed release of endogenous oxytocin and as oxytocin is almost certainly involved in the development of secure attachment in the baby, they may also risk under-stimulation of oxytocin-related behaviours at birth in both mother and baby with potential impact on the child's social development (Jonas *et al.* 2009).

The mothers were able either to lift their babies out of their bodies as they were being born, or to hold them immediately at birth and for as long as they wanted. To be the first person to touch their baby and to have prolonged and undisturbed contact with no pressure to examine, weigh or measure the baby was very much cherished by the women. It has been suggested that this first interaction between the mother and her baby may be a critical period in the development of the capacity for sociability (Odent 2010). Skin to skin contact and breastfeeding release oxytocin, decrease cortisol levels, lower blood pressure and promote a feeling of calm (Uvnäs-Moberg 2003). As Uvnäs-Moberg (2010) explains, babies have both food hunger and touch hunger. The monkeys in Harlow's classic 1950s experiments preferred the terry cloth mother-substitute to the wire mother, even though the latter was holding the bottle of milk. When frightened, the baby Rhesus monkeys always chose the terry cloth over the wire mother, suggesting that the need for touch is critically related to feeling secure.

Mia felt strongly that there was nothing more important than that she should hold her baby close after he was born, and she resisted any interference with this. Her behaviour instinctively recognized what has been called the 'sensitive period' immediately after birth, during which close contact between the mother and her baby may have a positive long-term effect on their interactions (Bystrova *et al.* 2009). The midwives had called the GP, without telling her:

> My GP came whom I don't know at all really. He didn't want to be there! He said, 'Could I just listen to baby's heart; could I just do the check now?' And because I was at home – and I would never have done this in any other circumstances – I said, 'Actually, he's just feeding now, so I don't want you to do that'. And the midwives were saying, 'But doctor really needs to do this' and I said, 'But he's only just been born'. And you know, the checks they do, they're horrible, they make the baby scream. And I thought that he'd just had quite a peaceful birth and they wanted me to give that up because of the GP whom I'd never asked for anyway. And I said, 'What's the worry? You can listen to his chest if you like, but not while he's feeding. I don't want to move him'. Everybody was visibly fed up with me for doing that but it was interesting that when I read my notes later, the GP had written, 'Full examination declined; mother and baby bonding', so he did respect and understand my decision.

There is increasing evidence to suggest that human health is constructed in the mother's womb. There may also be a critical period at birth when certain behaviours which prepare the baby to become a sociable human being are triggered by the release of oxytocin. What the mothers in this book realized instinctively is in the process of being confirmed by science. It may be wise, therefore, at this point in the development of the evidence-base, that stressful interventions in the antenatal, intrapartum or immediate postnatal period are kept to a minimum (Simkin 1986).

Key points

- There is almost certainly a link between the mother's stress levels during pregnancy and the physical and mental well-being of her child. Antenatal care does not yet acknowledge that the foetus might have a psychological and spiritual life which is developing concurrently with its organs.
- Women in the UK today tend to be isolated during pregnancy and breast-feeding, times at which they are especially in need of peer group contact and support.
- Under-stimulation of oxytocin-related behaviours at birth in mother and baby potentially impact on the child's social development.

References

Anderson T. (2002) Out of the laboratory: back to the darkened room. *MIDIRS Midwifery Digest*, 21(1):65–9.

Austin M., Leader L. and Reilly N. (2005) Prenatal stress, the hypothalamic–pituitary–adrenal axis, and fetal and infant neurobehaviour. *Early Human Development*, 81(11):917–26.

Bystrova K., Ivanova V., Edhborg M., Matthiesen A. S., Ransjö-Arvidson A. B., Mukhamedrakhimov R., Uvnäs-Moberg K. and Widström A. M. (2009) Early contact versus separation: effects on mother-infant interaction one year later. *Birth*, 36(2):97–109.

Egliston K. A., McMahon C. and Austin M. P. (2007) Stress in pregnancy and infant HPA axis function: conceptual and methodological issues relating to the use of salivary cortisol as an outcome measure. *Psychoneuroendocrinology*, 32(1):1–13.

Hodnett E. D., Gates S., Hofmeyr G. J. and Sakala C. (2007) Continuous support for women during childbirth. *Cochrane Database of Systematic Reviews*, Issue 3. Art. No.: CD003766. DOI: 10.1002/14651858.CD003766.pub2

Jonas K., Johansson L. M., Nissen E., Ejdeback M., Ransjo-Arvidson A. B. and Uvnäs-Moberg K. (2009) Effects of intrapartum oxytocin administration and epidural analgesia on the concentration of plasma oxytocin and prolactin, in response to suckling during the second day postpartum. *Breastfeeding Medicine*, 4(2):71–82.

O' Connor T., Heron J., Golding J., Beveridge M. and Glover V. (2002) Maternal antenatal anxiety and children's behavioural/emotional problems at 4 years: Report from the Avon Longitudinal Study of Parents and Children. *The British Journal of Psychiatry*, 180:502–8.

Odent M. (2004) *The Caesarian*. London: Free Association Books.

Odent M. (2007) *Birth and Breastfeeding: Rediscovering the needs of women during pregnancy*. East Sussex: Clairview Books.

Odent M. (2010) 'New criteria to evaluate the practices of obstetrics and midwifery.' International Conference on Birth and Primal Health, Gran Canaria, 28 February 2010.

Pascali-Bonaro D. and Kroeger M. (2004) Continuous female companionship during childbirth: a crucial resource in times of stress or calm. *Journal of Midwifery and Women's Health*, 49(4):19–27.

Selye H. (1982) History of the stress concept. In Goldberger L. and Breznitz S. (eds) *Handbook of Stress: Theoretical and Clinical Aspects*. New York: Free Press.

Shakespeare W. (1969) *Hamlet* (Edited by Rylands G.) Oxford: Clarendon Press (New Clarendon Shakespeare).

Simkin P. (1986) Stress, pain and catecholamines in labor: part 1: a review. *Birth*, 13(4):227–33.

Slade P. and Cree M. (2010) A psychological plan for perinatal care. *The Psychologist*, 23(3):194–7.

Talge N. M., Neal C. and Glover V. (2007) Antenatal maternal stress and long-term effects on child neurodevelopment: how and why? *Journal of Child Psychology and Psychiatry*, 48(3–4):245–61.

Tritten J. (2010) 'Roundtable discussion "childbirth in 2050"'. International Conference on Birth and Primal Health, Gran Canaria, 28 February 2010.

Uvnäs-Moberg (2003) *The Oxytocin Factor: Tapping the hormone of calm, love and healing* (translated by Roberta Francis). Cambridge, Massachusetts: Da Capo Press.

Uvnäs-Moberg (2010) 'Oxytocin: the inner guide to motherhood'. International Conference on Birth and Primal Health, Gran Canaria, 27 February 2010.

Verny T. R. and Weintraub P. (2002) *Tomorrow's Baby*. New York: Simon and Schuster.

Wadhwa P. D., Sandman C. A., Porto M., Dunkel-Schetter C. and Garite T. J. (1993) The association between prenatal stress and infant birth weight and gestational age at birth: a prospective investigation. *American Journal of Obstetrics and Gyaecology*, 169(4):858–65.

Websites

International Covenant on Economic, Social and Cultural Rights: www2.ohchr.org/english/law/cescr.htm (accessed 28 March 2010).

Jewish pregnancy: www.jewishpregnancy.org/spirituality_for_pregnancy/segulot.html (accessed 28 March 2010).

Pravda: http://english.pravda.ru/main/18/90/359/1560_childbirth.html (accessed 28 March 2010).

Science Daily: American Thoracic Society, 'Mother's prenatal stress predisposes their babies to asthma and allergy, study shows', Science Daily 19 May 2008: www.science daily.com /releases/2008/05/080518122143.htm (accessed 28 March 2010).

8　Men's experience of home birth against medical advice

The role of men in childbirth has been a topic of academic and popular debate for some time, raising strong feelings in fathers' organizations, among women and in the press. In 2009, the French obstetrician, Michel Odent, who has long opposed the presence of fathers in the delivery room, argued his case at the Royal College of Midwives' annual conference. Odent is not a lone voice amongst obstetricians in questioning the centrality of the role accorded to fathers on the twenty-first century labour ward. The work of Klaus and Kennel (1997) on support provided to women by women during labour concluded more than a decade ago that: 'The father's-to-be presence during labor and delivery is important to the mother and father, but it is the presence of the doula [another woman] that results in significant benefits in outcome'. Odent's views were hotly contested by members of the Fatherhood Institute, notably Adrienne Burgess who wrote in the *Guardian* that fathers' attendance at labour benefitted both mothers and babies (Burgess 2009). However, the most recent Cochrane Review (Hodnett *et al.* 2007) of support during labour concludes that women are best supported by other women during labour.

The fathers' role during the labours described in this book was often not a central one. This is not to suggest that men's knowledge of their partner isn't valuable; indeed, it can be crucial. Grace, whose positive pregnancy story is told briefly in the final chapter, recounted how her husband's intervention rescued a potentially difficult situation:

> I didn't have any urge to push and then the baby passed meconium and the midwives were concerned because they thought second stage should have been a lot quicker. So I think they were worrying about shoulder dystocia and they called an ambulance. But my husband who had been with me for my previous two births knew I needed to be much more upright, so he said, 'Come on, get up' because the midwives had tried to get me on my back and legs in the air. And as soon as I got my upper body upright, the baby came. I only needed two more pushes and he arrived before the ambulance did and was absolutely fine.
>
> Grace

Whatever their role during labour, the role of the men during their partners' pregnancies, and especially in the third trimester when relationships with health professionals became particularly fraught, was crucial.

The effect of quality partner support in reducing women's anxiety in pregnancy has been explored by Rini *et al.* (2006). These researchers studied 176 women's perceptions of the support provided to them by their partners and recorded reduced anxiety in the women from mid to late pregnancy if their perception of the support was favourable. Pajulo *et al.* (2001) found that partner support was especially powerful in affecting the woman's adjustment to her pregnancy, either for better or for worse, and much more powerful than the influence of other people who were close to her. In addition to psychological benefits of partner support, Hoffman and Hatch (1996) noted that intimate support from a near family member or partner seemed to enhance foetal growth, even for women whose life circumstances were not especially stressful.

The positive effect of support in enabling people to cope with challenges in everyday life, whether those associated with major life transitions such as becoming a parent, or with those arising out of difficult relationships, is generally accepted. The women in this book referred constantly to the support they received from their partner both in making the decision to have a home birth, and in sticking to that decision in the face of professional opposition. Lack of support from a partner has been found to be predictive of antenatal depression (Reid *et al.* 2009); in the case of the women in this book, it seems probable that it was the unfailing support of their partners that enabled them to retain positive mental health.

The men demonstrated genuine concern, listened to the women and expressed their strong feelings on their behalf both in private discussion at home and in encounters with health professionals. Leonie's partner's decision to support her was based on 'insider information' regarding hospital labour and birth. As a paramedic, he had seen birth in hospital and felt strongly that he did not want that kind of experience for his wife. Leonie described him as being more keen on her having a home birth than she was herself.

Other men were sometimes initially surprised by the woman's choice of a home birth, and some voiced concerns about its safety. Just as the women sought further information from books, the internet and health professionals to justify their decision to go ahead with a home birth, and also talked to members of their peer group of childbearing women, the fathers tended to do exactly the same. Maria-Sofie's partner experienced major reservations about her desire for a home birth, but once he had spoken to midwives and perhaps, more importantly, to other fathers whose partners had had a home birth, he was converted:

> The first time I said to him I thought I wanted a home birth, his immediate reaction was: 'Why do you want one of those?' And I said, 'Well, you will be sent home afterwards if I go into hospital and I will be on

my own and I won't have any support'. And his reaction was, 'But you might bleed to death at home'. So we went to the Home Birth Support Group and he talked to some other dads and there were a couple of independent midwives there and then he was happy about home birth. From that point, he was completely supportive with everything I have ever chosen to do in terms of pregnancy. We regularly have the Home Birth Group here now in the evening and he often sits in so that he can talk to the other dads about it.

This kind of 'conversion' experience was quite common; men who were at first worried by home birth became, sometimes very quickly, ardent supporters once they had spoken to people who had experienced it, either personally or in a professional capacity. There is scope for research into what aspects of other men's experiences of home birth impress expectant fathers most favourably and what information health professionals convey that reassures them effectively.

Alessia and her husband were strongly united in their determination to have their twins at home. Her husband accompanied her to every meeting with the consultant and senior midwives that took place towards the end of her pregnancy. It appears to have been presumed by the consultant that, as the father-to-be, he would be less than happy with the home birth decision and that he could be used to persuade Alessia to change her mind and agree to come into hospital for the births. The ethically questionable strategy of trying to drive a wedge between the couple did not escape their notice:

> She [the consultant] tried to play us off against each other. 'And what do you think about this?' she said to him as we were sitting there. 'Do you approve of this?' And he said, 'Well, I think there's nothing wrong with a home birth. Why shouldn't we have these babies at home?'

This father was particularly mistrustful of health professionals' motives for trying to persuade his partner to come into hospital. His negative perception of the maternity service appears to have been based on resistance to authority which he saw as being exerted simply for the sake of achieving conformity, and on his feeling that he and his partner were the victims of unfulfilled promises:

> Government policy says that you have choice. Maternity policy that the government released two years ago says that women should have the choice to give birth wherever and however they want, and yet this is obviously not being implemented. So what's the point really?

An identical sense of betrayal was voiced by one of the fathers interviewed in the Finnish study by Viisainen (2001). The researcher concluded that the father was deeply suspicious of a biomedically orientated maternity service, which he considered as capable of deceit to meet its aim of keeping all births within hospital walls (p. 1114).

Alessia's partner's concept of risk was far more pragmatic than that of health professionals. Extrapolating from experience in his own field of work, he felt that there were serious flaws in the risk arguments that were being put forward to him:

> There are always risks, but you can't plan for everything. As an engineer, I know that. If you build a retaining wall, there's always a chance it's going to fall down. There's always a chance that the building will fall down. But does that mean you never build a retaining wall? We wouldn't get anywhere, would we? If you applied the kind of philosophy they have now about home birth to the moon landing, we would never have got to the moon. You shouldn't, as a prospective parent, have to go through such an ordeal just because you want your children at home.

His case for the impossibility of achieving zero-risk is accepted by the Expert Group on Acute Maternity Services to the Scottish Executive (2002):

> Furthermore in assessing and apportioning levels of risk within maternity services it must be acknowledged and highlighted to women, that there is no such thing as 'zero' risk and that risk cannot be the same for every woman. While maternity care experts can measure risk and communicate estimated levels to individuals, this information is filtered and may reflect professional and social bias.
>
> (p. 1)

He fiercely resented the condescending way in which Alessia was spoken to by her consultant, and articulated his objection to staff's attempt to adopt a parental, supervisory role in relation to them when they were adults, not children, negotiating for a service:

> Alessia has got a degree and my profession is an engineer. We're both intelligent people and they speak to you like you're kids.

He felt that she knew her own body best, that she was the best person to judge her ability to birth these particular babies and that birth should be left to mothers:

> You should get all the men out of birth – every single one – because it's got nothing to do with men. Men can't ever give birth, so how can a man, however learned, however experienced, ever know what it's like?

This father had complete trust in his wife's strength to birth safely at home, a trust reflected in the attitudes and behaviour of the partners of the other women in this book. At a crisis point in her relationship with health professionals, Margret had the following discussion with her partner:

> I said, 'How would you feel if we just didn't ring them?' [when she was in labour] And he said, 'Well, if it's what you want to do, then I'll trust your judgement'.

He then had a moment of concern, and suggested:

> We could just ring them right at the very end and see how things are going.

When Margret voiced concern about having professionals attend her who did not have confidence in her, he reiterated that he was happy for her to do what she felt best:

> If that's what you want to do, fine.

One man, who was interviewed for this book because his story was particularly interesting, was a father who was also a general practitioner. Jon's own advice had been, at least initially, strongly against his wife having their baby at home:

> Lola said she would very much like to have her birth at home and that was a big difficulty for me to begin with because I'd always envisaged home birth as slightly hippy, a slightly crazy thing for women to do, and I certainly had no experience of home births among friends or family. I'd not even had patients request a home birth, but I had run over in my mind what I would say if they did and it would be, 'Well, if that's what you want to do, then so be it, but I really wouldn't recommend it'.

As happened with other men whose partners' stories are told in this book, the strength of Lola's belief that labour and birth are normal processes, requiring minimal assistance, convinced Jon that there was, indeed, no particular reason for her to be in hospital. Previous experience – again as is often the case in home birth decisions – was also influential. Both Lola and Jon had been in hospital as patients, and it was partly as a result of reflecting on how difficult he had found that experience that Jon agreed to the home birth:

> Both of us had had non-obstetric experience of being in hospital. People talk about the 'psychological undressing' of being a patient and it's absolutely true. It's one thing being ill and going through that, but being well and going through that for a normal process, that really made me reconsider my position on where the best place is to have a baby.

Lola's absolute confidence in her ability to give birth to her baby safely at home was such that Jon was quickly won over:

> So when I'd come to terms with it, which was rapid, then we didn't talk much more about it because it was a done deal; this was how it was going to be.

Like other men in the book, once the decision was taken, the logic of normality which he had learned from his partner, led him to assess the 'complications' which arose during her pregnancy differently from how he would have done previously:

> Between 32 and 34 weeks, Lola had her full blood count done which showed that she had a very borderline anaemia which is absolutely normal in pregnancy. We were informed by the midwives that a home birth would not be possible. And we could find no reason, no rationale.

Nonetheless, he was grateful for support from knowledgeable outsiders, just as the women in this book were when they encountered obstacles to their home birth plans. Support came from a mother who ran the local Home Birth Group and proved as important at this stage as it had to Erin's and Maria-Sofie's partners:

> It was around this time that I met someone from the Home Birth Support Group and she advised me about how we could challenge the local midwifery service and say, 'Actually, we don't really mind about the haemoglobin. We are still having a home birth and therefore we would still like you to bring round our home birth pack'.

The father's important role in providing support to his partner during pregnancy difficulties proved arduous and Jon found that having to argue their case 'added a lot of stress to the final part of the pregnancy'. Lola's haemoglobin level finally crept above the figure which enabled the midwives to feel able to support the home birth. Prior to this happening, however, the couple had decided that, if necessary, they would resist 'the system' by subverting it, as other couples in this book did:

> We were prepared to hold out on the haemoglobin, so if it had become an issue at the last minute, we were going to try to see how far we could get on our own at home, then ask the midwives to visit and then say that actually we weren't going into hospital.

The trajectory of Jon's experience of pursuing home birth against medical advice followed exactly the same course as that of many of the women (and presumably, their partners) in this book. His initial doubts about home birth were allayed as a result of discussion with his partner during which her confidence and determination reassured him. On encountering opposition from health professionals, he sought advice from someone experienced in supporting home birth couples. Finally, he participated in devising a strategy to subvert the system should it continue to resist a home birth on grounds that he considered inappropriate.

His experience during his partner's labour and birth also mirrored that of other men. When men attend antenatal classes to prepare them for birth in hospital, they are very concerned to find out what their role will be and how they can help their partners. They want to be 'involved' and not to feel superfluous during a labour which will be monitored and overseen by a variety of health professionals. Their partners are also concerned about what their men will be doing; much discussion focuses on how the men can help simply by ensuring that the woman is not left alone during labour.

Research has also explored the roles of men during labour. An early 'classification of roles' was devised by Chapman in 1992. She suggested that men assume one of three roles: that of coach, team-mate or witness, and that the most frequently adopted role is that of witness. In 1993, Chalmers and Wolman carried out a review of studies to find out whether fathers' support has an impact on the course of labour; they concluded that research has yielded contradictory findings, although most studies suggest that women do appear to value fathers' presence. Hallgreen *et al.* (1999) noted that the 11 men whom they interviewed found labour demanding and were disturbed by its unpredictability. Lili's description of her partner's experience of her labour bears this out:

> He suddenly found he was quite emotional throughout the birth, because I was doing it and he couldn't do anything. He was saying, 'I didn't think it would be like this. I didn't think it would be so long. I didn't think you'd be making so much noise and I didn't know it would be so difficult'.

This is exactly the picture painted by Johnson (2002), who carried out a series of twenty face-to-face interviews and reported that some of the men had felt under-prepared for the experience of labour. They had not been able to define a role for themselves and questioned whether they had had any purpose in being present. On reflection, they considered that they had experienced 'obligatory role adoption' in acquiescing to expectations that they would be present at the birth of their children. The study by Deave and Johnson (2008) in which another 20 fathers were interviewed demonstrated similar findings. The men's experience, related to the birth of their babies, had been one of anxiety, feeling excluded from what was happening, and surprise and concern at the length of labour.

All of these studies have been of men's experience of supporting their partners during labour and birth *in hospital*. Just as the clinical environment may distort women's instinctive responses to labour, so it is possible that it inhibits men from adopting a role, or a variety of roles, that they would find easier to manage than the 'coaching' or 'team-player' roles, or even the 'witness' role that they appear to take on in hospital. During the home births recounted in this book, the men tended to stay at a distance from the women, often not even in the same room. The women did not necessarily want them to remain close; in fact, they sometimes requested to be on their own.

The men tended to figure very little in the women's accounts of their labours. It would appear from their partners' accounts that they were able to decide on the degree of involvement in the labour that they wanted to have. Backström and Wahn (in press) identify the opportunity to make such a choice as correlating with men's satisfaction with their birth experience. Margret noted that she had spent a lovely day at home with her partner in early labour; at one point they had been out shopping together. Yet as soon as she started describing more intense labour, her partner dropped out of her account and the midwives came to the fore and it was the midwives who talked her through the panic she felt when she went into second stage:

> They really reassured me and mothered me and helped me through it.

This was very much a case of the mother needing mothering herself and turning to women experienced in birth to provide it. It is unclear in Margret's story whether her partner was in the room at this point or elsewhere.

The 'invisibility' of the men in the women's stories of their labours suggests that all the women needed was to know that their partners were at hand and would not be leaving. Given that they were present somewhere in the house, they did not often refer to their help and when they wanted support, it was generally to other women that they turned. Erin's partner massaged her during the first part of her labour, but it was the doula who made her feel safe:

> She knocked on the door and I stood up to say, 'Come in, the door's open' and my waters broke all over the floor and for me, that was perfect because she was there and things were starting to happen and it made sense because she made me feel safe.

Leonie describes the very strong relationship she had with her baby during labour and the unobtrusive presence of her midwife. However, she does not mention her partner until the baby is born:

> The midwife didn't really advise me at all during the birth apart from encouraging me to do what felt right for me and the baby. She occasion-ally would come with her doppler and listen to his heart rate; it was always strong and steady. The baby never panicked and I believe this was because I was constantly in touch with him in between those strong contractions and we were working together during them . . . he was very

blue when he was born which alarmed my husband but apparently this is normal. The midwife let the cord stop pulsating before my husband cut it.

Mette gave birth before her midwives arrived. While her husband was immensely caring, he could not provide the particular kind of reassurance and support that she needed as she came to the end of second stage:

> I was just rocking over the stool and every time my partner had a free moment, I was asking him to either rub my back or fill up the birth pool or get on with this and that. My waters had broken and the contractions were getting very intense and I couldn't really let him do anything else. I just thought, 'I think I need a midwife; I really can't do this any more' and I think it would have been very helpful to have someone around to say, 'It's OK; that's perfectly normal; you are about to have the baby'. Because I really didn't know what I was going to do; it just seemed to be too much.

Despite having medical knowledge and physically supporting his partner as she gave birth to their baby, Jon felt as helpless as Mette's partner probably did when the labour reached its crisis:

> Lola was between my legs and I have no idea how long we were in that position for. I think back and it's sort of stretched to infinity yet, at the same time, it was seconds. And suddenly I could hear the baby crying and then it was this absolute blur for the next five to ten minutes because there was so much going on and I just didn't know what to do. I think I was pretty much stuck to the spot and just thinking, 'Oh, what's going on? What's happening next?'

The men were busy (and apparently content) 'fetching and carrying'. Jon's account of the birth of his baby includes periods which were blurred in his memory, generally those when, from his point of view, there was not much happening, and those which were clearly focussed – times when he was active, as happened when his partner decided to give birth upstairs rather than downstairs:

> It was such an effort for her to get upstairs that there was no way she was coming back down. So there was a brief period when I had to ferry all the bits upstairs – the paediatric resuscitation kit, all the towels – so there was a dozen trips up and downstairs for this amazing array of equipment that had started to collect in different places.

The 'busy-ness' experienced by the men was, however, purposive and self-directed rather than determined by professionals or technology. This is in contrast to the way in which Lili described the role of her friend's partner in labour. In fact, one of the reasons Lili wanted a home birth was precisely to avoid reducing her partner to merely watching machines and giving her instructions. She felt that what her friend described as 'working together' was in fact meaningless:

> I was talking to my best friend who was saying how labour is and your husband is watching the screen and he's telling you when the contractions are coming and telling you when to push and that was good because then you knew how much gas and air you needed. And just listening to that made me think, surely that's not how it has to be?

Her concern that the kind of support provided by this father was dictated by machines and mechanical, and did not include the kind of physical and emotional support that she wanted, was also a concern of the men in Johnson's longitudinal study (2002a), which found high levels of stress among 53 fathers at the time of birth. This was especially so if the men felt under pressure to be present and anxious about fulfilling their 'role' because they were not clear what it was supposed to be. Johnson states that confusion remains as to the nature and purpose of men's presence during childbirth and speculates whether fathers who are surprised by the emotional burden of attending their partners in labour may be negatively affected in terms of bonding with their offspring.

The anxiety so often expressed by *women* in antenatal classes regarding the role of their partners in hospital was not experienced by the women in this book either during pregnancy or labour. In fact, the men were quite naturally 'looked after' by the midwives:

> It was great for my husband as well because I hadn't really thought about what he'd be doing. I was always thinking about how I was going to get the baby out and not about what he'd be doing. I think being at home made him feel so much more comfortable. The midwife was looking after him as well, and if she thought I needed to be on my own, she'd say, 'Oh, let's go and have a cup of tea' or whatever.

Lili

Lili's assertion that her partner's experience was enhanced by the individual support he received from the midwife is reflected in Chandler's and Field's study (1997), which reported that men found labour to be much harder work than they had anticipated and that they needed considerable support. The partners of the women in this book seemed to find a natural role for themselves in taking children to their grandparents to be looked after when the mother went into labour, filling the birthing pool, spreading shower curtains and towels on the floor and getting anything the midwife wanted. This sense that their partners were occupied and thereby 'involved' appears to have liberated the women to concentrate on their labours.

While none of the women in this book mentioned choosing a home birth so that their partner could have a particular role during their labour, many of them acknowledged that once the baby had been born, the presence of the father was an essential part of being a new family. Erin spoke about how she wanted to avoid the situation which arises in hospital when the father has to leave and go home after the birth of the baby:

> There was the issue of when the father gets sent home and I said to the midwife, 'I really don't fancy that; I think I'd just rather be with him and if I'm in hospital, that's not going to happen'.

An account given by a man following the home birth of his second child expresses the same idea from a father's point of view:

> At the end of a home birth, the midwives leave. Not you. This is the way it should be. In a hospital, you are torn away from your newborn child and your exhausted wife at the very peak of your emotional vulnerability.
> (Ven whose home birth featured in the TV series,
> 'Home Grown Babies')

Deave and Johnson (2008) discuss how the men in their study felt anxious and emotional at the time of the birth and had difficulty resolving their emotions because there was often no time allowed for them to be alone with their partners and babies.

Following the birth of his son, Jon was struck by how normal the experience of having a baby at home felt, and how quickly a completely new, but nonetheless very familiar, life took over again:

> It's such an amazing thing after the birth just to have time together in peace and quiet, in private. The midwives made us tea and they sat downstairs and did their paper work. They left at 10 o'clock and then we were by ourselves in a pristine house as if nothing had happened there the night before. I made the biggest breakfast I think either of us had ever eaten in our entire lives, which again was brilliant.

This combination of normality and celebration was keenly relished by the men. Lili described her partner's reactions in similar terms to Jon:

> We were sitting there, watching TV with the baby, and my partner was just saying, 'This is the most incredible moment' because he had his dressing gown on and the baby was snuggled up on his chest and we were just sitting there, watching TV. He said, 'It seems so normal'. It felt so completely normal for him; it was just like he was thinking, 'Here's my son; he's been born; we're bonding'. He was overawed by it really.

The women in this book felt strongly that they knew what was best for them, their babies and their families in terms of where they should give birth. The decision-making about place of birth was, in every case, primarily theirs. They had no difficulty in convincing their partners that their decision was rationale and would cater best for both his and their own physical and emotional needs. There is no indication from the women's stories that their partners' support weakened as they came into increasingly acrimonious contact with health professionals. Rather the opposite; resistance to patriarchal control, a determination to exercise the choice that the health service had promised them, and anger at the treatment of their partners provided increasingly strong motivation for the men to continue to resist the authority of medical knowledge (Viisainen 2001).

Key points

- Men who were at first worried by home birth became ardent supporters once they had spoken to people who had personal or professional experience of it.
- During the home births recounted in this book, the men were able to decide on the degree of involvement in the labour that they wanted to have rather than experiencing 'obligatory role adoption'.
- The men were busy during the labour but they were self-directed rather than directed by professionals or technology.
- The women were free to concentrate on their labours because their partners were occupied, 'involved' and looked after by the midwives.
- The combination of normality and celebration experienced at a home birth was deeply appreciated by the men.

References

Backström C. and Wahn H. (in press) Support during labour: first-time fathers' descriptions of requested and received support during the birth of their child. *Midwifery*.

Burgess A. (2009) Hard labour. The *Guardian*, 20 October, available online at: www.guardian.co.uk/commentisfree/2009/oct/20/childbirth-fathers-present-benefit (accessed 6 April 2010).

Chalmers B. and Wolman W. (1993) Social support in labor: a selective review. *Journal of Psychosomatic Obstetrics and Gynecology*, 14(1):1–15.

Chandler S. and Field P. A. (1997) Becoming a father: first time fathers' experience of labor and delivery. *Journal of Nurse-Midwifery*, 42(1):17–24.

Chapman L. (1992) Expectant fathers' roles during labor and childbirth. *Journal of Obstetric, Gynecologic and Neonatal Nursing*, 21(2):114–19.

Deave T. and Johnson D. (2008) The transition to parenthood: what does it mean for fathers? *Journal of Advanced Nursing*, 63(6):626–33.

Expert Group on Acute Maternity Services (2002) Reference report – section 5: risk assessment and management within maternity services. Report submitted to the

Scottish Executive Health Department, March, available online at: www.sehd.scot. nhs.uk/publications/egas/egas-02.htm (accessed 8 April 2010).

Hallgreen A., Kihlgren M., Forslin L. and Norberg A. (1999) Swedish fathers' involvement in and experiences of childbirth preparation and childbirth. *Midwifery*, 15(1):6–15.

Hodnett E. D., Gates S., Hofmeyr G. J. and Sakala C. (2007) Continuous support for women during childbirth. *Cochrane Database of Systematic Reviews* 2007, Issue 3.

Hoffman S, Hatch M. C. (1996) Stress, social support and pregnancy outcome: a reassessment based on recent research. *Paediatric and Perinatal Epidemiology*, 10(4):380–405.

Johnson M. (2002) An exploration of men's experience and role at childbirth. *The Journal of Men's Studies*, 10(2):165–82.

Johnson M. (2002a) The implications of unfulfilled expectations and perceived pressure to attend the birth on men's stress levels following birth attendance: a longitudinal study. *Journal of Psychosomatic Obstetrics and Gynecology*, 23(3):173–82.

Klaus M. H. and Kennell J. H. (1997) The doula: an essential ingredient of childbirth rediscovered. *Acta Paediatrica*, 8610):1034–6.

Pajulo M., Savonlahti E., Sourander A., Helenius H. and Piha J. (2001) Antenatal depression, substance dependency and social support. *Journal of Affective Disorders*, 65(1):9–17.

Reid H., Power M. and Cheshire K. (2009) Factors influencing antenatal depression, anxiety and stress. *British Journal of Midwifery*, 17(8):501–8.

Rini C., Schetter C. D., Hobel C. J., Glynn L. M. and Sandman C. A. (2006) Effective social support: antecedents and consequences of partner support during pregnancy. *Personal Relationships*, 13:207–29.

Viisainen K. (2001) Negotiating control and meaning: home birth as a self-constructed choice in Finland. *Social Science and Medicine*, 52:1109–121.

Websites

Burgess A. (2009) Hard labour. The *Guardian*, 20 October, available online at: www. guardian.co.uk/commentisfree/2009/oct/20/childbirth-fathers-present-benefit (accessed 6 April 2010).

Hodnett E. D., Gates S., Hofmeyr G. J. and Sakala C. (2007) Continuous support for women during childbirth. *Cochrane Database of Systematic Reviews* 2007, Issue 3. Art. No.: CD003766. DOI: 10.1002/14651858.CD003766.pub2 (accessed 6 April 2010).

Scottish Executive Health Department: www.sehd.scot.nhs.uk/publications/egas/ egas-02.htm (accessed 3 May 2010).

9 Free birth
The end of the choice continuum

Free birth or unattended birth excites fascinated, and often horrified, interest among the public, midwives and the media. It appears to many as an utterly nonsensical activity in a country and an age when maternity care is free, midwives are highly trained, obstetrics commands sophisticated technologies and hospitals are striving to provide more homely environments to enable women to relax and enjoy the birth of their babies. It is easy to dismiss women who choose free birth either in a kindly if patronizing manner as 'hippies' or in a less kind and more defensive manner as 'irresponsible'. Women who free birth their babies may stimulate genuine incredulity amongst other women, or may provoke them into justifying their own decision to have their babies in hospital. Such a defence often refers to the 'safety' of hospital, thereby claiming the moral high ground for the mother who presents herself as taking responsibility for the well-being of her baby by choosing a medical environment in which to give birth.

Women and health professionals who find free birthing challenges some and often all of their most cherished beliefs may be comforted by the fact that it is a minority activity. And so it is, but it is an activity undertaken by a significant and increasingly vocal minority. Nor are the reasons women decide to call no-one to attend their labours different from those of women who choose home birth against medical advice or perhaps even women who choose an 'allowed' home birth. They simply appear to trust their own knowledge of their bodies more than they trust the maternity care system.

Free birthing is the most extreme form of avoiding the system and thereby challenging it. It is undoubtedly a form of social protest, a means of expressing discontent with a publicly provided service (to which the women have contributed through their taxes) by fleeing from the service. Free-birthing women seek simply to side-step the kind of clashes with health professionals, which caused Leonie, for example, to leave every consultation with her doctors in tears, and especially to avoid distress in the late stages of pregnancy when women feel an urgent need to be 'nesting':

> The Supervisor of Midwives invited me to meet her, so I went in with my husband and my doula. I was very nervous and very big at this point

and kind of just wishing that I could get this issue sorted so that I could relax and get the house ready.

Erin

Viisainen's study (2001) of home birth amongst Finnish women includes one couple who chose free birth. This was both a personal choice that they felt was best for their family, but also a political act which they intended should influence others:

> They felt that their experiences have also initiated others to express discontent with the system although most are not ready to voice it and even less ready to act upon it.

(p. 1116)

Romaně, who gave birth to her first baby in hospital and who free-birthed her second, in fact shared many similarities with the other women whose stories are told in this book. Above all, she shared their conviction that her labour and birth would be normal and require no intervention. As with any profound belief, it is difficult to know why belief in their own childbearing capacity was so strong with these women and is apparently far less so for others. It would seem logical to presume that evolution has down the centuries required that women should trust in their ability to give birth. If fear generates adrenaline and adrenaline reduces oxytocin production, excessive fear of childbirth would be counterproductive in terms of perpetuating the species. Grantly Dick-Read (1944) inspired the British childbirth movement with the story of how he attended a young woman's birth in the East End of London. Amazed by her calm and the absence of any signs of distress through the most intense stages of labour, he later questioned her about her experience. The mother informed him that she had not known that childbirth was supposed to hurt. From this account, Dick-Read deduced that childbirth was not inherently painful, but became so when women's fear caused them to tense up (produce adrenaline), with the result that contractions became more painful and less effective.

Some of the home birth women in this book found labour very painful and some were surprised by how little pain they felt. None used any drugs to control pain. None of the women even mentioned the unavailability of major pain-relieving interventions at home as a drawback when discussing their home birth choice. Analgesia appears to have been irrelevant in the face of their self-belief. Romaně described how her 'instinctive decision' to free birth was based on her recognition that she 'could do this alone'. Mette also expressed her belief that birth is not supposed to be traumatic and should not be viewed as an event outside the normal physiological experience of women:

> I believed that birth could be good, that it could be a positive experience.

That doesn't seem like rocket science – yet birth is presented as a huge emotional, psychological obstacle that you have to overcome.

Romaně's choice to give birth to her second baby, unattended by a midwife, was underpinned by exactly the same reasons as those of the other women in this book who chose home birth against medical advice. This is an important observation because it suggests that free birth is not an activity happening in a parallel world to home birth, carried on by women whose thinking has nothing in common with that of other women. Romaně chose to challenge the system because she found that it could not and would not cater for the whole range of her needs in connection with having a baby. The logic of her thinking simply led her to an end-point that was further along the choice continuum than the other women progressed to. That it is a continuum is illustrated by Margret and Mia who, when pushed to the limit by the negativity of their encounters with the maternity service, both considered not calling a midwife to attend their labours.

By unravelling the strands of Romaně's decision-making, the similarities in her motivation to choose free birth to that of the other home-birthing women can clearly be seen. Her first labour had been difficult and unrewarding:

> The birth of our daughter was a traumatic experience.

She was frightened of experiencing another labour as painful and as unsatisfying as the first. Mia's motivation to have a home birth was similar. Her first baby had been born by caesarean following an induction which she had not wanted and several changes of shift as a result of which she had had no continuity of carer:

> I agreed to an induction, knowing that it wasn't what I wanted and I saw the midwives on three different shifts – that's how long it was. Thursday was when I went in, Thursday morning, and she was eventually born by caesarean on Saturday morning and I'd dilated to 9.5cms. So that was a caesarean birth and it was truly horrendous in every possible way; it was one of the worst days of my life.
>
> Mia

Romaně stressed the exposure of her first labour, both literal and metaphorical, the loss of privacy and the feeling of control being taken away from her:

> At the time of the birth, the midwife who came to our home totally disrespected the environment we'd created. We had a fire burning, candles lit, and I was dressed in a night gown. The midwife came in and turned on the lights and made me strip down.

Mette also referred to feeling demeaned by the treatment she had received during her first birth:

> There were two midwives whom I remember for the impact they had on me immediately after the birth. The things they said to me after the birth made me just want to throw them out of the house, they were so awful.

Romaně had gone into hospital to give birth to her first baby; her experience there led her to believe that there were pressures operating on staff that were outside of and irrelevant to what was happening in her labour:

> Eventually, we went into hospital, where I believe the whole thing was rushed because the midwife was keen to finish her shift on time.

This same concern that staff actions might sometimes be motivated by issues other than the welfare of mother and child was very strong with Mia also. She had read a letter in the notes for her first birth in which a consultant had expressed the opinion that it was possibly because of boredom on the part of staff that she had finally been delivered by caesarean.

Zadoroznyi (1999) describes the experience of childbirth as 'a critical reflexive moment in many women's lives' (p. 267). The women in this book who had given birth prior to the pregnancy in which they chose home birth against medical advice had reflected at length, and analyzed what they, as individuals, needed to ensure that the birth of their babies was a significant and positive rite of passage. Romaně and Mette identified that what had been missing from their first labours and what they were determined to have for their second, was a sense of ownership:

> What my partner and I had wanted was *a personal experience*, but we hadn't had that.
>
> Romaně

> It was like the whole experience was kind of ripped from me; you're just totally subject to what they think is best for you. And I know they have your interests at heart, but it feels very demoralizing and disempowering to be treated like that, especially when you are really determined to have *a positive experience that's your own.* [Author's emphasis]
>
> Mette

This is in accord with the extensive body of literature which, for at least the last 35 years, has explored factors influencing satisfaction with childbirth and has identified that the woman's sense of being 'in control' is a significant positive predictor of her assessment of the quality of her labour and birth experience. In 1975, Willmuth, a psychiatrist, noted the importance for labouring women of 'maintaining control'. In the twenty-first century, Goodman *et al.* (2004) again highlighted 'personal control' as critical. Eileen Hodnett has produced several papers which have reported an inverse relationship between anxiety in labour and perception of control (Hodnett and Simmons-Tropea 1987) and which have identified 'involvement in decision-making' (Hodnett 2002) as one of the key factors influencing positive evaluations by women of their labours.

Between her first and second pregnancies, Romaně and her partner came to the conclusion that they needed to free birth in order to achieve a birth that would have meaning for them:

> We wanted the birth to be as intimate as possible and to be the first people to touch our baby, but we were told by the midwife that this wasn't a possibility. In the end, at 40 weeks, we announced that we wanted to have an unassisted home birth.

Lea and her partner chose home birth because they, too, felt that the hospital environment and hospital staff could not give them what they wanted:

> My husband and I spoke about it and decided that the only way we could get a natural birth and the water birth that I wanted was to have the baby at home. And along with that was our thinking about having an independent midwife because I had read that a lot of women who have home births end up going into hospital because the midwives practise under hospital policy and that encourages them to transfer you very quickly.

Romaně wanted to determine her own behaviour in labour, and felt that if she were attended by midwives, hospital policies and attitudes would prevail, negating the conditions which had led her to choose a home birth in the first place. Margret chose an independent midwife because she, too, feared that staff from within the maternity service would expect and perhaps insist on her having a certain kind of labour:

> I wanted a home birth and the benefits of home birth. I didn't want a hospital birth at home which is what they were offering me. I didn't want to have to battle when I was in labour for the birth that I wanted.

Romaně felt that it was essential that she have the maximum of privacy during her labour. She considered that any outsider, including midwives, would threaten this:

> We needed to delve deep into ourselves. Having another presence at the delivery was never going to work for us; any amount of observation would inevitably inhibit our ability to birth naturally.

Although midwives were in attendance for Mia's labour, she felt instinctively that her labour would progress better if she was alone:

> I said, 'Can I be by myself now?' And everybody went out. I knew I would probably be best by myself. I didn't like the expectation of being watched by people. I had a lot of time alone.

'Being watched' is one of the conditions that Odent identifies as inimical to normally progressing labour. He writes that, 'Since humans are mammals . . . physiological considerations suggest that in order to give birth women must feel secure, without feeling observed' (www.wombecology.com). For Romaně, the presence anywhere in her home of professionals who are trained to *observe* would compromise the environment which she wanted to create to enable her labour to happen easily.

Despite her assertion that her decision to free birth was 'instinctive', Romaně nonetheless felt the need, as did the other women in this book, to seek support from a peer group and from carrying out her own researches. This is a critical feature of the stories of all the women; while determined to challenge the system and to assume responsibility for their pregnancies and births, they needed to know that they were not alone in their beliefs and to find reassurance that the actions they intended to take had already been taken by others:

> It's only really through reading other people's birth stories and tapping into communities of women online who have had similar experiences and experienced similar discrimination that I managed to achieve the birth I wanted.
>
> Erin

The language used on free-birthing websites is reflected in both Romaně's account of her philosophy of birth and that of the other women in this book. The premises which are put forward to support free birth by activists such as Shanley (1994) are that childbirth is not a disease, that birth should be peaceful, that it should reinforce the woman's autonomy and give her an appreciation of the power of her body to bring babies into the world. Women do not need to be told what to do during labour; they already know. Home birth with a midwife in attendance is merely to transport the medical model of birth from the hospital into the private domain. Often considered the guru of unattended birthing, Shanley writes on her website, www.unassistedchildbirth.com:

> This site is based on the belief that childbirth is inherently safe and relatively painless provided we don't live in poverty, and do not interfere either physically or psychologically. Drugs, machinery, and medical personnel are not only unnecessary in most cases, they are also no match for a woman's own intellect and intuition.

Romanĕ's interview reflected the 'spiritual' language found on some of the free-birthing websites; she spoke of birth as:

> . . . an open celebration of our love and an understanding that we can totally surrender to and trust each other, my body and our baby.

Mette also had a philosophy of birth and argued that:

> A good god cannot condemn half the race to agony in childbirth; it doesn't make sense.

On a site called Childbirth Solutions, advocating unassisted birth, Lana Kutarna writes:

> The mother is equipped from conception with the tools necessary to look out for herself during pregnancy and to birth well . . . I therefore question whether the standards of obstetrical and midwifery care are really in our best interests or in the best interests of our babies.

Alessia's birth philosophy was very similar to this; her confidence to choose home birth was based on the evidence of centuries of successful childbearing by the females of the human race:

> I kept coming back to the same idea and the same belief that this was right for us and millions of women in the past; they managed to do it without the great intervention of hospitals. So surely I should be able to try and give birth to our babies at home. I knew lots of reasons why things go wrong when women go into hospital; when you get scared, things go wrong and then intervention happens.

Whatever the popular imagination may presume that women who choose to free birth are doing while they are in labour, the way in which Romanĕ managed her labour was, in fact, identical to what Leonie and other of the home birth women had found helpful:

> When my waters broke and the contractions started, I just really chilled out and had a nap. Then I had some juice and went for a walk. By the evening, the contractions had become stronger and I had another lie down. I started using vowel sounds to ease the contractions.
>
> Romanĕ

> We had a good plate of scrambled eggs on toast and headed for a long walk along the river to let gravity help the process along. We got home and by 7pm, the contractions were more regular . . . I began to vocalize and it helped me relax.
>
> Leonie

The only significant difference in Leonie's account of her labour is that there was no point at which she had a discussion with her partner about when to call the midwife. This decision was prominent in all the other stories in this book.

Romaně described her unassisted birth as 'healing', by which she seems to have meant that it helped her to resolve doubts about herself which her first traumatic experience of birth in hospital had raised. Mia felt the same, stating that as a result of the way in which her third child was born, she felt 'restored', and Mette spoke at length about the psychological impact of her home birth:

> It definitely helped me forget the emotional trauma and redeemed it in a way; it's like overcoming adversity and being rewarded for believing that it could be a good experience.

Following her free birth, Romaně, along with many of the home birth women, felt more confident and competent to mother her child than she had done with her first baby:

> My daughter, who is now 14 months old, and I have a fantastic relationship; it's amazing how different it is to the one I have with my other child, who is now five years old.

Margret analyzed the possible impact on women's confidence to mother when pregnancy and birth are highly controlled:

> If your instincts as a mother are not respected during pregnancy, it really undermines you from the start. I do understand why so many mums go to books now instead of thinking, 'Well, I'm a mum and millions of women have been mothers before me without books!' Of course they'll reach for books because they are so used to being told that the way their bodies are working is wrong and so, how can they trust their instincts? How do you parent your baby when everything else has been controlled for you?

At the time of my speaking to Romaně, she was pregnant with her third child and planning another unassisted birth. There is no statutory obligation for a woman in childbirth to call a midwife or doctor; it is legal for a woman to deliver her own baby.

While the number of women in the UK today who are choosing to free birth is almost certainly very small, Beverley Beech (2000), militant Chair of the Association for Improvement in Maternity Services, feels that that number may grow if women sense that the choices they are being offered around care in pregnancy and labour are, in fact, more limited than the rhetoric of a personal, woman-centred maternity service would imply:

> I received another call yesterday from a woman in the west country who informed me that she is so dismayed with the sub standard maternity care she is receiving she is going to birth at home unattended . . . We know of a number of women who have deliberately birthed at home unattended and others who intend to do so.

Free birthing, as social protest, is unsettling both for those who administer and provide the service that is being protested against, and for those continuing to use the service, even when service-users vastly outnumber dissenters. One defence against such protest is to dismiss those involved in it as a reckless minority, or to accuse them of being irrational, or perhaps to portray them as having immoral or even criminal tendencies. Indeed, the possibility that there may be cause for legal action against free-birthing women has already been raised. One NHS doctor, blogging under a pseudonym, has suggested that women could be sued by their (damaged) offspring for having had a home birth, let alone an unattended one (reported by Groskop 2007).

It nonetheless seems unlikely that free birthing will disappear in the near future, and certainly not while the maternity service is confronting women who request home birth with 'tiny hoops to jump through, held high and always moving' (Mia). When 'avoidance protest' becomes a phenomenon, it is worthy of attention. Labelling women who choose free birth as deviants will, as is always the case when such an approach is used to counter opposition, merely strengthen the commitment and influence of those who choose the disallowed choice.

Rather than simply ignoring the protest, dismissing it, or blindly attacking it, a more intelligent approach might be to examine the protesters' case and analyze whether there is merit in any of the arguments they are raising. By confronting protest in this way, it may be possible to reform the system so that those who are currently choosing to remain outside it can be brought inside, with benefits for both parties and loss of self-esteem for neither. Free birthing may be seen as the realm of women who are unable to appreciate the benefits of a biomedical technocracy underpinned by hard intellectual evidence, or it may be seen as providing an opportunity for the maternity service to have a reflective pause. The trans-national nature of childbirth protest, with free birthing emerging simultaneously as a phenomenon in the United States as well as in Europe, suggests that its influence may develop beyond the periphery currently occupied by highly motivated activists.

Acknowledgement

This chapter is based on a telephone interview with Romaně and also on an interview given to Charlotte Philby for the *Independent on Saturday Magazine* (11 July 2009).

Key points

- Free birthing is a form of social protest. Discontent with a publicly provided service is expressed by refusing to use the service.
- Free-birthing women avoid the maternity service because it does not cater for the whole range of their needs in connection with having a baby.
- They seek to avoid the loss of privacy and control which they associate with being observed by a health professional, and which they feel will compromise their labours.
- Labelling free-birthing women as deviants is likely to strengthen the commitment and influence of the women who choose it.
- The free birthing phenomenon provides an opportunity for the maternity service to reflect on whether it is meeting women's needs as comprehensively as it can.

References

Beech B. (2000) A nail in the coffin for home birth. *AIMS Journal*, 12(3), available online at www.aims.org.uk/Journal/Vol12No3/ukcc.htm (accessed 10 April 2010).

Dick-Read G. (1944) *Childbirth Without Fear: the principles and practice of natural childbirth*. London: Harper and Brothers.

Goodman P., Mackey M. C. and Tavakoli A. (2004) Factors related to childbirth satisfaction. *Journal of Advanced Nursing*, 46(2):212–9.

Groskop V. (2007) Going it alone. The *Guardian*, 9 May.

Hodnett E. (2002) Pain and women's satisfaction with the experience of childbirth: a systematic review. *American Journal of Obstetrics and Gynecology*, 86(5):S160-S172.

Hodnett E. D. and Simmons-Tropea D. A. (1987) The Labor agentry scale: psychometric properties of an instrument measuring control during childbirth. *Research in Nursing and Health*, 10(5):301–10.

Shanley L. Kaplan (1994) *Unassisted Childbirth*. Westport CA: Bergin and Gravey.

Viisainen K. (2001) Negotiating control and meaning: home birth as a self-constructed choice in Finland. *Social Science and Medicine*, 52:1109–121.

Willmuth L. R. (1975) Prepared childbirth and the concept of control. *Journal of Obstetric, Gynaecologic and Neonatal Nursing*, 4(5):38–41.

Zadoroznyi M. (1999) Social class, social selves and social control in childbirth. *Sociology of Health and Illness*, 21(3):267–89.

Websites

Childbirth Solutions: www.childbirthsolutions.com/articles/pregnancy/unassistedbirth/index.php (accessed 9 April 2010).

Michel Odent: www.wombecology.com/physiological.html (accessed 8 April 2010).

Unassisted childbirth: www.unassistedchildbirth.com/ (accessed 9 April 2010).

10 Advocacy, empathy and autonomy

The women whose stories are told in this book were exceptionally courageous. They made difficult choices, reflected on them when challenged, discussed them with others, researched them and, after they had reached the conclusion that they were still the right choices for them, they were prepared to put their heads above the parapet and defend them. Fighting their corner was emotionally and physically draining, however, and what all the women were hoping to find, and initially expecting to find, was an advocate within the maternity service. They sought an advocate who would support them in their choice to give birth at home simply because it was *their choice*, regardless of whether the professional herself considered it to be right or wrong.

The challenges for professionals and health care managers of offering women choice in maternity care have been almost exclusively formulated as challenges to do with availability – availability of different locations of care so that women can choose point of access; availability of a range of practitioners so that they can choose by whom they would prefer to be treated; availability of different kinds of pregnancy and birth technologies for them to choose between. The most difficult aspect of the provision of choice, however, lies elsewhere – it is in supporting women who make choices that it was never intended or foreseen that they would make.

Robinson (2007) notes that there are professionals who do not understand that informed consent cannot exist without its opposite. There remains an assumption that if people have approached health care services, and have received information about the treatment which staff feel is best for them, they will consent to it. The logic of informed refusal is that some patients want simply to find out what treatment would involve and then assess for themselves whether its associated risks, indignities, surrender of control and potential outcomes make it preferable to having no treatment or to having a different kind of treatment, perhaps outside the health service.

The maternity service has found it very difficult to accept that women may access the service, find out what it has to offer, look at its practices, judge its successes and its failures, and decide that they don't want what's on offer. Professionals may find it difficult to separate rejection of their service from a feeling of being rejected themselves; it is irritating and disturbing when others do not place the same value on an opinion, treatment or service as you do yourself. Some women may put forward a view of the maternity service which is very challenging to professionals, even if, within their peer group, doctors and midwives might accept its accuracy:

> There are lots of cases where things have gone wrong because the medical profession has intervened and caused problems, but it's always dressed up as, 'Oh well, it's a good job we were there because if not, you would have died'.
>
> Alessia

The conundrum of choice, therefore, is whether all and every choice can be 'allowed', provided that it is within the law. And if a choice is currently legal, but not supported by health professionals, should it be put outside the law? While home birth is not illegal in this or any other country in Europe, it *is* illegal in the UK for someone to assist a woman at a home birth if that person is not registered as a midwife. This has led free-birthing women to send their partners out of the house while they give birth, for fear that they might be prosecuted (Nolan 2008). If making it illegal for anyone other than a maternity professional to assist at birth is an attempt to enforce conformity and persuade women to consent to the attendance of a midwife, it is ironic that its consequences may well be to add to the perceived dangers of free birthing by depriving women of all support.

If making a choice in health care genuinely means freedom to choose among legal alternatives, it seems both unreasonable and offensive to indicate by word or action or 'tone' that some choices are considered inappropriate, regrettable or stupid (a word used by Lili's midwives in relation to her decision not to be induced at 42 weeks). Indeed, the United Kingdom Central Council for Nursing and Midwifery, before it became the Nursing and Midwifery Council, stated that a recognized midwifery role is to provide support *if a patient refuses treatment or care* (UKCC 1996). While lawyers may argue that some patients cannot be considered to have decision-making capacity, it is quite evident from the fluency of the women in this book, from their ability to mount and defend their arguments, that they were rational and that the hostility they provoked was founded on antipathy to patients who do not share health care professionals' view of their situation.

The most striking feature of the stories told in this book is the women's failure to find advocates among public sector maternity professionals:

> I just bolstered myself with my own resources. I knew I was not going to get anything from the NHS to support me.
>
> Mia

They could not find staff who respected and accepted their choice because it was *their* choice and it was informed, and who would support it and them in the face of opposition:

> So I was just really, really looking for someone who might really be able to support me.

They rarely found professional friends, or were able to form relationships based on trust. As a result, their confidence in themselves as childbearing women and as mothers was impaired and they suffered from a diminished sense of both physical and psychological well-being (chapter 3).

The occasions on which the women met staff who did indeed see choice as the woman's prerogative and who were prepared to support her, were singled out for special mention:

> [The consultant] was very honest, she didn't try to scare me at all, she was brilliant. She said there was a very small risk that I was going to have a shoulder dystocia and it would happen in hospital as much as at home and she said, 'The decision's yours really'.
>
> Margret

What the women craved was care which made them feel strong, confident and safe. Contrast the way in which Erin described a meeting with the Supervisor of Midwives:

> . . . she tried every tactic she could to psychologically break me down;

with her succinct and grateful summary of her relationship with the doula she employed:

> . . . she made me feel safe.

At a time of major transition in their lives, women are looking constantly for affirmation and encouragement, especially with a first pregnancy when they are preparing for a rite of passage which is, for most, extremely anxiety-provoking:

> She only ever made me feel fantastic about myself and the pregnancy and she gave me faith in myself and my instincts.
>
> Leonie

Simply by making Leonie feel good about herself, her midwife was rewarded with her trust and appreciation. Many of the women identified how important it was for them in preparing mentally for the birth to receive positive affirmations from others:

I need people who believe in me and feel I'm competent enough to give birth.

Margret

They contrasted scaremongering:

. . . they kept putting doubts in my mind;

Margret

with the way in which the attitude of some staff made them feel strong and relaxed:

. . . and she was very matter of fact about it and she said, 'There's nothing to worry about'. And I thought, 'Well why aren't all the other midwives like this?'

Margret

There is an urgent need for a cultural shift, a shift from a negative paradigm of birth which is accurately captured by 'reality' television, particularly in America, to a positive paradigm based on the assumption that labour will be a normal event. The women were seeking advocates whose concept of birth was not the familiar one portrayed in the first quotation, but rather the one that was familiar 50 years ago, portrayed in the second:

In 'Maternity Ward,' no laboring women are depicted out of bed. Whether they are in early labor or pushing, they are flat on their backs. Machinery is everywhere. Blood pressure cuffs are on; electronic fetal monitors are strapped onto bellies. Legs are draped, and support people are off to the side. Heart-racing music plays whenever something 'dramatic' happens. The mothers look terrified. I don't blame them. Within five minutes of watching the show, I am terrified for them.

(Lothian 2003)

I have stated on numerous occasions that there is no more need to interfere with the course of normally progressing labour than there is to tamper with good digestion, normal respiration and adequate circulation.

(Montgomery 1958)

Many of the women understood that it was difficult for midwives to challenge the policies of the Trust by which they were employed and that there might be implications for their future employment should they do so. However, they still felt that staff should, at the very least, be able to demonstrate an 'advocacy of empathy' by showing understanding of the woman's feelings:

I've met loads of midwives who don't seem to understand the strength of feeling a woman can have. They don't understand the depth of feeling and that it is actually quite rational [to want a home birth] because the risks to your mental state, to your emotional state of going through such a traumatic hospital birth again are catastrophic, so the relative risk of whatever they think could go wrong doesn't seem as bad.

Mia

The women wanted staff to put to one side their learned 'professional' response to what they were asking for, and to try to understand the experiences and the emotions that were informing their choices. They sought holistic, woman-centred care rather than an approach to their 'case' based on the management of disease (Alderdice 2010):

I just thought she'd be really encouraging of someone wanting a positive experience second time around after having had such a bad time.

Mette

Fear is very powerful as a motivating force. While creating fear of future disasters that might occur should they insist on birthing at home was employed as a means of dissuading women from their choice, the fear stemming from *previous* experience was often far more influential for the women:

I couldn't go back to the hospital where my daughter was born; I found it hard to even drive past it.

The women needed advocacy based on acknowledgement of the fear borne out of lived experiences, rather than coercion based on professionals' fear of events which might never happen.

Fear that staff did not understand or sympathize with their need to have a home birth led the women to mistrust them, and fear of the choice the women were making dulled the 'affective awareness' (Hunter and Deery 2009) of staff. The women felt that if they were to entrust themselves to the care of staff, staff must in turn trust their expertise – expertise based on previous experience of birthing, instinct, knowledge of their own bodies, and knowledge of the baby they were carrying.

In the 1960s, in a famous experiment conducted in an American school, Robert Rosenthal demonstrated that students will conform to the expectations that teachers have of them. A few years earlier, a Professor of Sociology at Columbia University, Robert Merton, had published *Social Theory and Social Structure* (1957), in which he described the 'self-fulfilling prophecy'. This entailed a false definition of a situation, leading to new behaviour which makes the original false conception come true. The self-fulfilling prophecy is a phenomenon that can be used to achieve positive outcomes as well as negative, an insight that has long been recognized in mental health care. From the founding of The Retreat in York in 1792, one of the earliest institutions providing humane care for the mentally ill, it has been a maxim in mental health nursing that sufferers are helped to recover if those caring for them *believe that they are able to do so* (Nolan 2000). This is closely linked to the principles of salutogenesis as previously discussed in chapter 4, namely that by showing someone the resources they possess to become well or achieve better health, and building their self-esteem to choose a health-promoting direction of travel, they can manage their own lives. By contrast, the twenty-first century maternity service appears to be perversely determined to send out the strongest possible messages to women that they are *not* able to birth their babies except under close surveillance and with considerable medical assistance. Perhaps it is not therefore surprising that intervention rates are increasing, as women live up to this relentlessly negative assessment of their essential female physiology.

The conditions of the self-fulfilling prophecy are that certain expectations are formed either by individuals, by services or by entire communities, of other people or of events. These expectations are communicated both subtly by tone of communication and non-verbal signals, and overtly by words and phrases that imply a particular direction of travel (e.g. the mother will 'be delivered', thereby implying that she will be passive in her own labour). These cues are picked up by people and affect their behaviour with the result that expectations become reality.

Having high expectations of people tends to make them perform better, and low expectations will have the opposite effect. It might therefore be suggested that if staff expect a woman to have a straightforward labour, she is more likely to do so than if they expect that there will be complications along the way. The struggle for normality has to take place in the minds and hearts of both staff and women. At the moment, because the philosophy and practice of biomedical positivism is so deeply entrenched, the maternity service is not capable of addressing escalating intervention and costs. By word and deed, it undermines women's belief in themselves, thereby reducing the incidence of inexpensive vaginal birth. The women in this book wanted normal birth; they believed themselves capable of it and were prepared to fight for it. It might have been assumed that they would find many friends among midwives whose profession is dependent on and committed to normality.

The maternity service struggles to understand the choices that some women make because the 'evidence' that it expects women to draw on to make their choices is uni-dimensional. The evidence drawn on by the women in this book was far richer and more varied than that presented to them by health care staff. Wickham (www.withwoman.co.uk) argues for there being many kinds of evidence, including the woman's and the midwife's intuition, women's experience, midwifery experience, research, the individual life experience of the woman and of the midwife, embodied knowledge, physiology, common sense and finally, policy and practice. Midwifery is ideally aware of all of these, rather than dominated and controlled by any single one. Page (1996) has estimated that only a very few of the decisions that need to be made in midwifery can be based on research evidence, and Kirkham *et al.* (2002) advise that the concepts underpinning midwifery and the policies which guide it should be kept constantly under scrutiny as knowledge advances. When practice is driven solely by policy and protocol, it is experienced by women (and by professionals) as tyrannical, insensitive, uncreative and demeaning of both women's and professionals' expertise. Women find that their own assessment of their situation, and the grounds on which they lay claim to expertise, are not respected and that they are not truly invited to make choices. Margret was able to evaluate the long-term impact of belittling women's understandings:

> I did feel very much that my opinions and my instinct – after all, it was my fourth pregnancy – weren't respected. If they are not respecting how you feel, your instinct as a mother, it doesn't bode very well for the rest of the pregnancy and the labour and also early parenting.

Rather than reducing women's respect for and appreciation of the skills of staff, the women in this book reserved the highest praise for staff who acknowledged their expertise in birth. In a passage full of gratitude for the care provided by her independent midwife, Maria-Sofie describes how the midwife affirmed her understanding of the stage of labour she had reached:

> I said to the midwife, 'I think I need to push' and she said, 'Well, if you think you need to push, then you are probably nearly there because you have done this before'.

It is hard to see what purpose is served by suggesting to women that they are not capable of giving birth, or how frightening them will lead to better outcomes. Gould (2004) suggests that the mark of good midwifery care is the ability to inspire trust and confidence in the birth process. There is sufficient evidence now to show that women who are frightened in labour, who cannot work with their bodies to make contractions effective, are likely to have difficulties in birthing their babies. It would therefore seem to make more sense in any terms that might be considered important by health service monitors and managers – be it reducing costs, improving the patient experience, freeing theatre space – if staff helped women to feel as capable as they can of achieving normal birth, in the expectation that such a positive attitude will of itself increase the chances of normality.

Normality is the preserve of the midwifery profession. The role of the midwife is to promote normal birth (International Confederation of Midwives 2005). Advocating for and protecting normal birth gives the profession legitimacy, credibility and purpose. Without a commitment to normality, there is no reason to have midwives. If birth is believed to be pathological, then staff with a background in pathology should logically take responsibility for the care of labouring women. Such staff could be nurses, trained in caring for those afflicted with ill health and disease, or obstetricians who specialize in abnormal birth. It would therefore seem to be in the best interests of the midwifery profession to support every woman who wants to achieve a normal birth. However, several of the women in this book expressed concern about midwives' commitment to normal birth and about the increasingly narrow parameters of midwifery practice. There is a challenge for the midwifery profession in these women's cogent analysis of what is 'wrong':

> Where birth is concerned and pregnancy, it's so over-medicalized that midwives have lost the ability to trust that most women can do it without medical intervention, without it being a highly medicalized event.
>
> Alessia

Perhaps such views should be dismissed as belonging to people who are outside the profession and who therefore lack understanding of the complexity of contemporary health services. However, it remains unsettling that one woman could comment, after numerous meetings with midwives at all levels, that speaking to a hypnobirthing teacher

> was *the first time* I'd ever spoken to anyone involved in the birth arena who just seemed to have no problems with birth. [Author's emphasis]
>
> Mette

All of the women felt that health staff were often practising in accordance with Trust policies and protocols, rather than autonomously making decisions based on their professional assessment of each woman's unique circumstances and needs. Nervousness about keeping within Trust policy over-rode the commitment of midwives at all levels of the maternity service to facilitating the choices of the women in their care:

> They didn't want me to follow what I actually wanted. They wanted me to follow their procedures.
>
> Margret

The women also noted that midwives seemed to be saying to them that they could do very little to help if their situation was anything other than that of a woman who had no previous medical or obstetric problems, who was pregnant with a single baby in a cephalic presentation, and who was choosing to give birth in hospital. Beech (2001) has highlighted a loss of confidence in midwives around normal birth. She finds it ironic that often when midwives receive extra training to expand their sphere of practice, the aim is not to enable them to learn new skills to safeguard normal birth even more effectively, but to learn skills to detect and remedy pathology. She construes the acquisition of such skills – ultrasound monitoring, ventouse delivery, for example – not as a development of the role of the midwife but as moving the midwife into a different realm of practice entirely. Alessia was able to summarize the same ideas very succinctly from the point of view of a woman who has given birth to six babies on five occasions and taken both an emotional and an analytical interest in the midwifery profession:

> The midwifery profession has changed so much from, well certainly 50 years ago. Midwives 50 years ago would go to women in labour and they would be able to deal with breech, they would be able to deal with twins. They would be able to do the things they are not able to do now. We were shocked to find that midwives are not allowed to externally manipulate the baby if the baby goes transverse, for example. Why aren't there midwives who can do ECV and deliver twins and breech babies? They are not allowed to use their common sense in dealing with situations that are outside the very very small box that is now considered the norm in their practice. And it really shocked me and made me feel cross for the midwives that they are so restricted.
>
> Alessia

The location of skills once familiar to all midwives *outside* the statutory maternity service should cause concern to the midwifery profession. Women who choose home birth against medical advice are likely to seek help from independent midwives because:

> Many independent midwives are experienced in helping women to give birth to breech babies, or to twins, or where a woman has had a precious caesarean birth.
>
> (Midwives Information and Resource Service
> 2008, 4)

The women in this book felt that there could often have been a 'common-sense' approach to their care, which was overlooked. Alessia describes how the solution to her desire to have a home birth for her twins was quite simple:

> If you put together a midwife who is experienced with twin birth vaginally and a midwife very used to home birth – with the two of them, we would be able to do it.

It was Erin herself, rather than the maternity service, who defined a common sense solution to her situation:

> I asked them to provide me with a new midwife who was pro home birth, who was experienced in water birth, and who could therefore support me

in my choices . . . we got a new midwife. She was fantastic, had delivered all her grandchildren at her daughter's home, very pro home birth, very experienced and very down to earth. Just what we needed.

The women expected that 'common sense' would be an essential attribute of midwives whose profession is to support other women having babies. When they came across it, they felt increased confidence and trust in their care:

> She was a very wise midwife and a very down to earth midwife; she had lots of common sense and we trusted her.
>
> Alessia

When in labour, the women valued particular attributes in their attendants, and certain key skills. They wanted a calm environment and a calming connection with their midwife, a connection which was underpinned by the midwife's previously declared and continually demonstrated confidence in the woman. The women's need for privacy was pre-eminent and they wanted their midwives to be able to sense when this need was best served by staying quietly close to them, and when it required them to be outside the room in which the woman was labouring:

> I spent a lot of time in the pool on my own which again was great because I knew there were people there and I knew I was being monitored, but I had my music on, I had some candles. It was all very dark and I felt fine throughout.
>
> Lili

The women were keenly aware that the flow of their labour could be interrupted and were critical of midwives who did not appear to understand how the 'shy hormone' (Odent 2010), oxytocin, works, and that the conversation the woman needed to have was with herself and not with other people:

> A few hours in and I was really into it. I wasn't totally aware of what was going on; I was really focussed. And the midwives came in and I didn't think they did very well by me. They were very talkative and interrupting.
>
> Mette

Odent (2010) considers the origins of midwifery to be in the role of the female relative who protected the labouring woman from the outside world – be that animal predators or human interference. When midwives did not recognize this as their role, the women became distressed and angry and had to provide privacy for themselves rather than having it provided for them:

I remember her trying to take my blood pressure while I was having a contraction. And another thing, during the labour, she came in to give me a tablet. I asked, 'What's this tablet for?' And she said, 'It's just a tablet we would like you to take'. And I am sort of saying 'Why?' I got quite annoyed and at one point, I said, 'I'm just going out for a minute'.

> Mia

By contrast, midwives who were able to sit back and let the woman labour at her own pace, who were able to 'drink tea intelligently' (Anderson quoted by Duff 2008), remaining watchful but not interfering, were highly valued:

They were very 'hands off'. They just let me get on with it; they didn't measure how dilated I was, or anything like that. They just let me get on with it.

> Lili

The women noted, probably because it was behaviour very different from what they would have expected to happen in hospital, that clock-watching did not appear to influence the behaviour of the midwives whom they considered the most skilled:

I never felt under any pressure; I didn't know what time it was or how long this had been going on, but I didn't feel under any pressure to do anything.

> Lili

When I wanted to get out of the pool, they all mothered me and wrapped me in towels and sat me on the settee . . . No one rushed me to make any movements and it was really nice.

> Margret

Women valued being given permission to do what felt right for them. Following their own instincts, and receiving support in doing so from a maternity care professional, appeared to be a winning combination in terms of easing labour:

I said to my midwife, 'When can I get into the birth pool?' And she said, 'Margret, you can get in the birth pool whenever you want'.

> Margret

I was saying to the midwife, 'I'm quite self conscious' and she said, 'Well do whatever you feel is right; if you want to wear stuff, do; if you don't, don't'.

> Leonie

Given privacy and support to do whatever felt right for them, the women were able to manage even very long labours well. They required little more of their midwives than occasional reassurance and encouragement:

> She'd been reassuring me the whole way, and it was just a bit of continuity really and I had eye contact with her and that continuing care while I was in the pool.
>
> Margret

> The midwife didn't advise me at all during the birth apart from encouraging me to do what felt right for me.
>
> Leonie

Particular skills excited the admiration of both the women and their partners, but they were not 'technical' skills (although clearly based on an excellent understanding of the structure of the pelvis and the physiology of labour); they were skills of working with the woman's body to help it give birth more easily:

> She'd move me into various positions and I'd been leaning on the stairs and then sitting on the loo and leaning over the loo and then sort of leaning over the pool. And then she said to me, 'Look, lie here, just have a bit of a sleep' and I think I slept for about half an hour.
>
> Lili

This understanding, both intuitive and learned, of how to assist labour, has characterized midwifery from the earliest centuries for which there are records:

> When the patient feels the throws coming, she should walk easily in her Chamber and then again lie down, keep her self warm, rest her self and then stir again, till she feels the Waters coming down and the Womb to open. Let her not lie long a Bed, yet she may lie sometimes and sleep to strengthen her, and to abate pain.
>
> (Jane Sharp 1671, *The Midwives Book*)

Skills which were at the opposite end of the spectrum from those associated with the technological and pharmacological management of labour attracted particular attention:

> Every time his position was changing with the contractions, he was becoming unsettled. And she did this bizarre thing of asking Lola to walk up and down the stairs sideways and it worked. I've never ever come across that before and I can't imagine that would have been an intervention done in hospital.
>
> Jon

After the injection, still nothing happened so one of the midwives asked my husband to go and get a beer bottle and got me to blow, to actually blow into it to make a tune. She got me doing this and I could feel the placenta moving very very gently, very very slightly, this slightly muffled movement. And all of a sudden, it shot out. I don't know if it was the injection, but I really believe it was the bottle blowing business.

Lea

There was a moment of concern when the baby didn't start breathing. The midwife didn't panic; she practised the Moro reflex on her and it worked instantly.

Alessia

The ultimate accolade given to the competent, sensitive and holistic midwifery practitioner was that she could facilitate an everyday event as if it was an everyday event:

I stood up, delivered the placenta, and the midwife caught it in a bed pan. She dried me off. I got out of the pool, went upstairs and got into bed, and that's where I breastfed the baby. And that was that really. She was fine, I was fine, I'm still breastfeeding three months later and I didn't have any stitches, I didn't have any problems.

Erin

The conditions for an excellent partnership between women and midwives, as illustrated in the women's stories, were shared faith in physiological birth, an empathic relationship based on the needs of the individual woman as opposed to an institutional relationship governed by generic protocols, and courage on the part of midwives to stand outside the status quo. Wagner (1999) has noted that the autonomy of midwives is dependent on the autonomy of women and the autonomy of women is dependent on the autonomy of midwives. The women in this book chose to exercise their autonomy by making a choice that was outside the menu of choices apparently available in the maternity service today. The midwives whom they valued were self-directing, able to make decisions informed by professional expertise, intuition and common sense. In order to create the conditions for a partnership of care, the women needed to meet health professionals who were as able to demonstrate autonomy in their practice as the women were in their choice of place of birth.

Key points

- The most difficult aspect of providing choice is supporting women who make choices that it was never intended that they would make.

- The conundrum of choice is whether all and every choice should be 'allowed'.
- Women feel that staff should be able to demonstrate an 'advocacy of empathy' by showing understanding of the woman's feelings.
- It is not surprising that intervention rates are increasing as women live up to the relentlessly negative assessment of their ability to give birth.
- It is hard to see how frightening women will lead to better birth outcomes.
- The location of skills once familiar to all midwives *outside* the maternity service should cause concern to the midwifery profession.
- The ultimate accolade given to the midwife is that she can facilitate an everyday event as if it is an everyday event.

References

Alderdice F. (2010) It's the person that counts. *Midwives*, December 2009/January 2010:34–35.

Beech B. (2001) Supporting the mother: where are the midwife advocates? *AIMS Journal*, 13(1).

Duff E. (2008) Passionate midwifery: a conference to celebrate the life and work of Tricia Anderson, available at www.iolanthe.org/Duff_Passionate_Midwifery_Sept08.pdf (accessed 13 April 2010).

Gould D. (2004) Trust me, I am a midwife. *British Journal of Midwifery*, 12(1):44.

Hunter B. and Deery R. (2009) (eds) *Emotions in Midwifery and Reproduction*. Basingstoke: Palgrave Macmillan.

International Confederation of Midwives (2005) 'Definition of the midwife'. Council Meeting, 19 July, Brisbane, Australia.

Kirkham M., Stapleton H., Curtis P. and Thomas G. (2002) Stereotyping as a professional defence mechanism. *British Journal of Midwifery*, 10(9):549–52.

Lothian J. A. (2003) 'Reality' birth: marketing fear to childbearing women. *The Journal of Perinatal Education*, 12(2):vi–viii.

Merton R. K. (1957) *Social Theory and Social Structure*. London: Free Press.

Midwives Information and Resource Service (2008) Where will you have your baby? *Informed Choice Leaflet 10*. Bristol: MIDIRS in collaboration with the Centre for Reviews and Dissemination.

Montgomery T. (1958) Physiologic considerations in labor and the puerperium. *American Journal of Obstetrics and Gynecology*, October.

Nolan M. (2008) Free birthing: why on earth would women choose it? *The Practising Midwife*, 11(6):16.

Nolan P. (2000) *A History of Mental Health Nursing*. London: Stanley Thornes Publishers.

Odent M. (2010) Oxytocin as the 'shy hormone', available at: www.midirs.org/development/MIDIRSEssence.nsf/ (accessed 13 April 2010).

Page L. (1996) The backlash against evidence-based care. *Birth*, 23(4):191–2.

Robinson J. (2007) Post traumatic stress disorder. *AIMS Journal*, 19(1).

Sharp J. (1999) *The Midwives Book: or the whole art of midwifry discovered* (Hobby E., ed.). Oxford: Oxford University Press.

UKCC (1996) *Guidelines for Professional Practice*. London: UKCC.
Wagner M. (1999) Through Irish eyes. *Midwifery Matters*, (83): Winter.

Websites

Duff E. (2008) Passionate midwifery: a conference to celebrate the life and work of Tricia Anderson, available online at www.iolanthe.org/Duff_Passionate_Midwifery_Sept08.pdf (accessed 13 April 2010).
Odent M. (2010) Oxytocin as the 'shy hormone': www.midirs.org/development/MIDIRSEssence.nsf/link/81B0FC4867DC184A8025768200528739?Open Document (accessed 13 April 2010).
Wagner M. (1999) Through Irish Eyes. *Midwifery Matters*, (83): Winter: www.midwifery.org.uk/irisheyes.htm (accessed 13 April 2010).
Wickham S. (undated) Evidence-informed midwifery 1: what is evidence-informed midwifery? www.withwoman.co.uk/contents/evidence/evidencemt1.html (accessed 12 April 2010).

11 The dialectic between possibilities and limits

There is no difficulty in bridging the gulf between the rhetoric of informed choice and the reality of practice, when women choose the choices that health professionals are confident to facilitate and which services are configured to meet. The stories in this book, however, suggest that the choice rhetoric is hollow when women make choices that conflict with the strongly held opinions of health professionals and the comfortable scope of routine clinical practice. There is nothing to suggest in previous chapters that the maternity service and those who work for it hold anything other than the best intentions when providing care for women, but it is nonetheless apparent that best intentions may sometimes be experienced by women as unkind, insensitive and unresponsive to their needs.

Maternity Matters (2007) stresses that the government's agenda is focussed especially on vulnerable families, by which the Report appears to mean families disadvantaged for such reasons as poverty, unemployment, difficulties in speaking English or experiencing domestic violence. However, it might also be suggested that women can be 'vulnerable' because they are considered to be at obstetrically 'high-risk'. As such, the government requires that extra efforts should be made 'to enable pregnancy and birth to be as safe and satisfying as possible for both mother and baby and to support [them] to have a confident start to family life' (DH 2007: 6). The conundrum is that stringent efforts were indeed made to try to keep the women in this book and their babies safe, but these efforts drove the women away from the maternity service and were perceived by them to be hostile to the goal of a satisfying birth and a confident start to family life.

It is, of course, right to acknowledge that there are women, supposedly 'at risk', who experience a common-sense response to the case that they put forward for a home birth, and enjoy embracing, confident and sensitive care from their midwives:

> When I went to book with the midwife, I was nearly 42 years old, and I said I would like to have a home birth because I'd had two previous ones with no problems. And the midwife said, 'Oh, we've had someone far older than you who's just had a home birth. That's absolutely fine'.

So she made me feel confident. But I had to go through a list of medical problems and if you'd had more than two on the list, you were supposed to see a consultant obstetrician. I ticked three of the boxes – two previous miscarriages, postnatal depression and over 37 – but I thought, 'None of these has any relevance to this pregnancy'. And when the Supervisor of Midwives saw the boxes I had ticked, I was expecting her to say, 'We'll book you in to see the consultant', but she didn't. She just said, 'Well, this pregnancy is fine and there's nothing here that's relevant. If anything does occur, we'll refer you, but at the moment, everything is fine'. So I never saw the consultant.

Grace

She describes how relaxed her pregnancy was:

I had shared care with my GP and at our surgery, when you go as a new patient, they give you a leaflet which says that the surgery does not support home birth because of the distance to the hospital. But my GP never queried my home birth. I made it quite clear that I knew what I wanted and I had confident midwives to support me because that's what their job is – as the advocate for the woman and not the advocate for the system.

Grace

Grace's calm assurance that she knew what was best for her and her family was met with an equally calm and mature response from her midwives, and her pregnancy was a series of encounters which had positive sequelae for everyone concerned.

The rhetoric of health policy states that 'maternity services must be planned to address current challenges' (DH 2007: 6), but does not perhaps recognize the challenges that are created when a highly controlling health service attempts to deliver choice hidebound by individual Trusts' policies and protocols. On the one hand, choice and democracy are comfortable companions, and also sit comfortably with professional autonomy; on the other, none of the three appears to be comfortable when trying to express itself in a maternity service that will not (or cannot) tolerate certain choices, is hierarchical and restrictive of the autonomy of non-medical staff. The maternity service therefore faces a dilemma in aligning its policies and practices with the rhetoric of choice. If the service wishes to set limits on choice, or cannot avoid so doing, then in the interests of transparency, the limits should be made clear to service users.

Arguments used by maternity care professionals when they oppose home birth may be based on assessment of physical risk alone. Using criteria of maternal and neonatal death and morbidity, there is no evidence to show that home birth is less 'safe' for *low-risk women* than hospital birth. Olsen's and Jewell's review for the Cochrane Database (2000) found 'no strong evidence to favour either planned hospital birth or planned home birth for low risk pregnant women', a position reiterated by the Royal College of Midwives:

> There is inadequate evidence for demonstrating hospital birth as the safer option for low-risk women.
>
> (Houghton *et al.*, 2008)

The women in this book, however, were labelled as 'high-risk' by staff, although low-risk by themselves. As Pilley Edwards (2005) has shown in her careful analysis of women's reason for choosing home birth, women's assessments of the risks around labour and birth take into account many more factors than the biomedical model allows. The women felt that the advantages of home birth summarized in the MIDIRS Informed Choice leaflet, 'Where will you have your baby?' outweighed the perceived risks of their not being in a medical environment:

> Research has shown that, compared to women giving birth in hospital, women giving birth at home used less pain relief, experienced fewer birth interventions, were more likely to be assisted by a midwife they knew and were also more likely to feel relaxed, in control and safe. This feeling of control is linked to better emotional outcomes for women.
>
> (p. 6)

All of the women had straightforward labours and gave birth to healthy infants. There are a number of possible explanations for this, all of which are worthy of reflection. Firstly, it may be that the women were not, in fact, high-risk and that whatever risk factors they were considered to have by staff were less significant than imagined. Secondly, home as the environment of birth may have been highly effective in calming tensions, promoting oxytocin release and thereby enabling the women to labour easily. Thirdly, it may be that the women themselves were the agents of their own safety, that their strong belief in their ability to birth their babies, based on the extensive research they had undertaken into their 'conditions', coupled with their emotional commitment to achieving a straightforward birth, over-rode any potential pathologies. Angela Horn, who moderates the most influential home birth website in the UK, writes:

> Sometimes it's hard to tell whether it is home birth which gets the good results, or the women who choose home birth.
>
> (www.homebirth.org.uk)

Professional understanding of childbirth lags far behind the complexities that cutting edge research is now presenting to us on an almost daily basis. To take a very simple example: a typical hospital birth for high-risk women involves induction with a syntocinon drip; continuous electronic foetal monitoring with two belts strapped to the abdomen; restriction of the woman to bed, control of the labour by midwifery and medical staff and almost inevitable sidelining of the woman's birth partner. There is little or no capacity for the woman to be touched other than for clinical purposes. Yet physiologists are demonstrating that one of the most effective ways of boosting oxytocin levels and therefore maximizing the efficiency of labour, is through:

> a combination of stimuli such as warmth, touch, massage, rhythmic motion and supportive and friendly psychological feedback.
>
> (Uvnäs Moberg 2003: 126)

Labour is a psycho-physiological event, not merely a physiological one, and it is this understanding which was so acute in the women whose stories are told in this book and which the maternity service did not recognize. Current professional practice often engages with just one of the multiple dimensions of labour and birth, and does not yet allow for the possibility that the way in which a woman gives birth will impact her ability to mother for not just hours after the baby is born, but for years. The 'maternity episode' is not complete at six weeks post delivery; it may never be complete, since the episode may have lifetime repercussions for the mental and physical well-being of both mother and child.

Government rhetoric is, in fact, shifting in the direction of accommodating increased understanding of the complexity of pregnancy and childbirth and of their long-term impact on the mother's self-perception, on her relationship with significant others, and on foetal programming, brain development and the ability of the child to cope with stress throughout life:

> Good maternal health and high quality maternity care throughout pregnancy and after birth can have a marked effect on the health and life chances of newborn babies, on the healthy development of children and upon their resilience to problems later in life.
>
> (DH 2007: 2)

The National Service Framework for Children, Young People and Maternity Services (DH 2004) is clear that promoting women's experience of choice and control in childbirth is significant in determining not just the mother's well-being, but also her child's.

Midwives, and to a lesser extent, doctors, were seen by the women in this book as in service to the service, rather than as in service to women. Bullying and coercion resulted when the letter of the law became of greater importance than the spirit (Romans 2:29). The women's stories raise particular issues for senior midwifery managers whose perceived role as Trust and maternity service 'agents' appeared sometimes to exclude both advocacy and even empathy. Without leaders who are able to demonstrate autonomous practice and the courage to take independent decisions, it is unlikely that clinicians in more junior positions will assume responsibility to accommodate 'different' choices. Employee turnover enables people to be brought into the service who fit the leaders' image, and to discourage those who prefer greater autonomy. The self-fulfilling prophecy is at work here – if staff are expected to work as their leaders do, they will do so. They may even lose the capacity to critically evaluate the service they are providing or see it as anything other than being as good as it gets in the best of all possible worlds:

> The following day, I had a midwife appointment with a community midwife and she was very flippant about my concerns and basically said, 'Well, we have to have guidelines'.
>
> Margret

The women's stories present uncertainty on the part of the service about the extent to which it should be fostering dependence rather than independence on the part of both maternity care staff and maternity care users. Yet new paradigms of care invoke, and emphasis on clients' strengths and potentials rather than their deficits, seek to help clients draw on internal motivation rather than imposing motivation from outside, and advocate that professionals should connect emotionally with clients, learn with them and work with them, rather than advising and directing them. Instead of deciding the care agenda for the client, post-modernist professionals seek to construct the agenda with the client; they expect to bring services to clients rather than focussing on how to bring clients to services. Paradigms of care for the next decade will aim to enhance social capital by enabling each individual who has contact with the health service to become a health ambassador to her community.

Creating dependence rather than independence allows the service to protect women from making 'wrong' choices because all decisions can be put in the hands of staff. This perpetuates paternalism (Gould 2004) and is not in the spirit of government documents which support the creation of a critical mass of well-informed health care consumers able to choose freely among options and make the decisions that are best for them. It is, in any case, inappropriate to try to protect adults from their own choices. On the contrary, it is a right of maturity that adults, as opposed to children, are able to experience both making choices and the consequences of those choices. The rationale for acknowledging the maturity of adult service users in health care is twofold; firstly, that it is unreasonable to presume to know what is right for competent adults better than they do themselves; and secondly, that understanding is only achieved when cause and effect can be clearly linked. The maternity service has a strong tendency to infantilize the mothers and families who access it, even though removing personal responsibility is counterproductive in terms of educating service users about the possibilities and the limits of health care. Creating dependence among *staff* is an attempt on the part of the service to protect itself from litigation by ensuring that policies and procedures which may not be appropriate in the case of each and every service user, but which will provide the basis for a defence in court, are adhered to. The benefits of fostering independence in both users and staff, which include greater satisfaction with the service on the part of women, greater job satisfaction on the part of staff who were, after all, trained to be autonomous practitioners, and greater possibilities for restructuring the service so as to meet more of the needs of more of the women who use it, are currently seen as less desirable than the perceived benefits of control through creating dependence.

The issues raised by the women's stories for practising midwives are fundamental because they are concerned with how they can protect their particular territory which is the territory of normality. There is consensus among professional and lay groups that promoting normal birth is the most effective way of honouring its physical and emotional complexity. The Maternity Care Working Party (2007) states that it is concerned:

> about rising intervention rates . . . as these procedures are known to be associated with both physical and psychological morbidity . . . we all want mothers and babies to come through birth healthy and well-prepared for the changes, demands and emotional growth that follow.
>
> (p. 1)

The analysis in the previous chapter of what the women were hoping that their home birth would give them, namely privacy, quiet, non-interference, personal control, and a meaningful transition to motherhood, requires consideration. Do contemporary maternity care environments come anywhere close to providing conditions which can accommodate the physical, emotional and spiritual aspects of birth, which the women recognized as critical? Is the 'architecture of compassion' (Foucault 2001) evident in the infrastructure of the maternity service? Mette decided that the only place which might provide that compassionate architecture was her own home:

> I did consider the hospital; it wasn't that I totally ruled it out. It's just that I knew that if I really wanted to be in a place of power and decision-making, the only place would be at home.

Walsh (2006) has described the kind of midwifery that the women were seeking as 'relational, "being" care' rather than 'task-orientated, "doing" care' (p. 1330). The women in this book knew that midwifery was in flight from itself when presenting in the way that they had sometimes experienced it:

> I think midwives do a fantastic job *when they do what a midwife should do*, but I think women are going to stop turning to midwives when they hear stories about birth. Why would they want a midwife when the fear is that they might get bullied into doing something that they don't want to do? I know a lot of midwives who wouldn't dream of treating women the way that I was treated and it does a great disservice to those midwives when their colleagues make women feel the way that I was made to feel.
>
> Margret

The promotion, protection and defence of normal birth falls within the remit of the midwife, and midwifery must protect women's rite of passage into motherhood. Women universally, in my experience, recognize labour and birth as key events in their lives, and while they protect themselves from a sense of failure by (correctly) flagging up how difficult normal birth is to achieve within the contemporary maternity service, the evidence suggests strongly that they are more satisfied with their birth experience, form a stronger relationship with their baby, and feel mentally more healthy following a birth with little or no intervention. Rites of passage are common across the world and respond to fundamental human needs. For the rite to be significant and thereby fulfil its purpose of marking a transition from one stage of life to another, the subject of the rite must have a *personal* experience. Birth may be the most significant rite of passage in a woman's life, and the creation of an environment which enables her to experience it as a personal journey is important. Some women may find that the hospital environment is not incompatible with this, although rates of postnatal depression suggest that it does not provide the sense of personal achievement that is the essence of a rite of passage.

The women had an overwhelming need for a rite of passage. They recognized this need and were surprised when health professionals did not. They also recognized the need to 'play the game' and provide the kind of evidence for their choices that the maternity service appears to value most highly. They therefore read widely and found their evidence. It may be that their use of the literature could be attacked on the grounds either that they did not understand the studies they were reading, or that they selected only studies which confirmed their point of view. Stewart (2001) however, accuses health professionals of exactly the same strategy, namely, welcoming evidence which maintains their control over clients (such as that supporting active management of labour), while rejecting other evidence which, by extension, supports more equal partnerships (such as the safety of home birth). Rather than becoming defensive, it may be a more intelligent and productive approach to ask why women who wish to make a choice that they are able to present as rational, human and natural, should be met with opposition and hostility.

It is too easy to categorize the women whose stories are told here as 'difficult customers' whom it was impossible to please. This kind of labelling attempts to shift responsibility from the health professional to the woman, to avoid entering into negotiations with her so that responsibility can be shared. Kirkham *et al.* (2002) have noted that:

> If the problem is identified as residing within the client, then change must come from the individual rather than from the system of care.
>
> (p. 550)

Labelling sidesteps the issues that 'difficult customers' raise; it consigns both the maternity service and midwifery to stagnation at best and to terrorism

at worst. Staff have to decide whether the constraints that are currently preventing them from coming alongside women are organizational or personal
constraints. Few would deny that midwives are constantly being asked to
help women make informed choices 'within a competing set of health service
agendas' (Hindley and Thomson 2005), on the one hand the medical agenda
of active management of pregnancy and birth, and on the other hand, the
agendas of women-centred care and normal birth. Martin (2007) has noted
that there is a dilemma which is perhaps felt nowhere so acutely as in the
maternity service (although it *is* felt in other specialities) between giving
control to patients as required by government policy and being 'an allegiant
member of a hierarchical structure that imposes rules, policies, protocols
and administers sanctions for failure to comply' (p. 13). Nonetheless, if the
midwifery profession cannot quickly and clearly define and establish its own
agenda, it runs the risk of becoming 'silent and complicit in the mistreatment
of birthing women and their partners' (Weston 2005). Hunter *et al.* (2008)
have noted that the context in which care is given – the context of exaggerated
risk management, fear of litigation, control of midwifery by obstetrics, mistrust and sometimes contempt for women's own understandings – seriously
impedes the formation of meaningful relationships between women and
midwives. The stories told in this book reveal an unacceptable picture of
unkindness, harassment, bullying and deceit, resulting in one woman making
the extraordinary statement that:

> I decided I wasn't going to call the midwives because I felt so so much
> more relaxed and happier and content knowing that they weren't going
> to come.
>
>   Mette

The women whose stories are told in this book were doubtless perceived
as unreasonable and objectionable by at least some of the staff whom they
encountered. Hostile treatment of women who refuse to tow the line has been
a theme in both academic research and in reports coming from the voluntary
sector for decades, making it difficult to dismiss. Green (1998) found that
women with very strong views irritated staff, and Robinson (2002), from
the Association for the Improvement in Maternity Services, has described
cruel treatment of women whose ideas about the kind of birth they wanted
were too challenging. That there is such a theme must be a wake-up call for
a profession that prides itself on 'being with' women and on inspiring trust in
families. Over twenty years before Gilbert (2009) examined the neurophysi-
ological impact of non-constructive criticism on an individual's sense of safety,
Flint had offered the same insights in *Sensitive Midwifery* (1986), where she
described how negative 'throw-away' comments ('your baby's very big'; 'your
baby's very small') could influence the woman's confidence and well-being
during the vulnerable period of pregnancy and early parenting.

If language does indeed construct reality, the language of pregnancy and birth is currently constructing a terrifying reality for childbearing women in the UK, and there is an urgent need for new metaphors to convey a different story about the journey to motherhood:

> I signed up for a hypnobirthing course, which was good; it was trying to positively reframe the way you think about birth. It fed into my whole mental preparation.
>
> Mette

The 'whole mental preparation' of the pregnant woman requires a discourse with health professionals which is carried on in language other than the merely biomedical. Pregnancy is complex; it is a time of transition when psychological, emotional, economic and social factors join together in new and challenging ways. It is a brief period of time, but it is fraught with opportunities which need to be presented to the mother as both positive and within her power to control.

I have heard it said that women who want childbirth to be 'an experience' are demonstrating both selfishness and superficiality in a world where half a million women a year die at some point along the pregnancy, labour and birth continuum and many others are glad merely to have survived. This is a mistaken representation and understanding of the genuine aspirations of women. A 'good birth' is rightly an end in itself because it contributes to women's sense that they are biologically and emotionally competent to birth their babies and this, in turn, increases their confidence in their ability and eagerness to mother their offspring well.

Pregnancy is life-changing; at present, it is oppressed by the relentless round of antenatal tests and examinations, restrictions and admonitions,

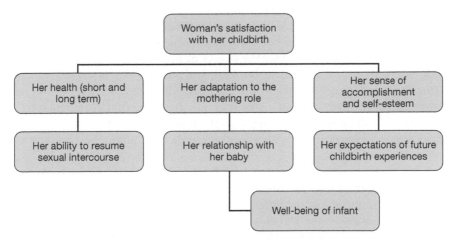

Figure 11.1 Links between a woman's experience of childbirth and future physical, psychological and social outcomes (based on Goodman *et al.* 2004: 213).

transforming it from a positive experience based on a sense of multiple possibilities into a negative one which does not allow for – indeed, seems to convey disapproval of – simple enjoyment of this exciting transition. It has become unlikely that many women living in the developed world are able to experience stress-free pregnancy. Yet increasing understanding of the negative effects of stress on the unborn baby will surely make such a situation unacceptable as we move into the second decade of the twenty-first century and take fully into account the:

> significant body of evidence from independent prospective studies that if a mother is stressed while pregnant, her child is substantially more likely to have emotional or cognitive problems, including an increased risk of attentional deficit/hyperactivity, anxiety, and language delay. These findings are independent of effects due to maternal postnatal depression and anxiety.
>
> (Talge *et al.* 2007)

The link between antenatal anxiety and postnatal depression is established, with antenatal anxiety being considered a frequent occurrence and increasing the likelihood of postnatal depression (Heron *et al.* 2004). The negative effects of postnatal depression on the development of a healthy and sustaining relationship between mother and baby have been well known for years (e.g. Murray and Cooper 1996; Murray *et al.* 1999; Hay *et al.* 2003).

Very very few women will choose home birth against medical advice. At present, very few women choose home birth even if they are considered to be low-risk. In the UK, the rate of home birth was 2.7 per cent in 2008 (www.birthchoiceuk.com). Once that figure rises to 5 per cent, however, statisticians consider that the rate will increase more sharply than in recent years (Dodwell 2009). This is because a rate of 5 per cent makes it likely that a pregnant woman who comes into contact with 20 other women expecting a baby or who have just had a baby will meet someone who is planning or has experienced a home birth. Once the stories of birth told by women are set in a different environment from the hospital, and are told in a different language from the language of obstetric complications, what are currently considered 'alternative' choices will become increasingly mainstream (Viisainen 2001). Lili said that she intended to 'sing from the roof tops about home birth' and Erin was working actively with a local midwife to promote home birth:

> It's very important to me to tell my story again and again because I think it can change birthing outcomes for other women. Once I'd had my baby, our pro-home midwife said to us, 'Can I give you this woman's number because she wants to talk to someone who's had a home birth and she's really up against it because she's getting near to 42 weeks?' So that started me getting phone calls, being given people's numbers by midwives.

A partnership between women and midwives may be the most effective way to bring about a cultural shift that will obviate the need for women to be bullied into compliance with protocols which they have had no part in devising and which are only fractionally responsive to their individual needs. Stapleton *et al.* (2002) note that 'a response that is woman-centred can only be made in alliance with service-users' (p. 610).

We are at a point of opportunity, when the 'cautious dialectic between possibilities and limits' (Anderson 2010) may be progressed to include more possibilities and less rigid limits. For professionals and women who do not care to envisage a future maternity service in which the definition of straightforward vaginal birth encompasses induction, epidural and assisted delivery – any combination of any interventions that results in birth of the baby by the vagina – and where women are infantilized and their basic biological function pathologized, this is a critical moment for action. Enkin *et al.* (2006) argue that we are now leaving behind the positivistic certainty of evidence-based obstetrics and moving into a new phase, carrying new possibilities, of 'reluctant but comforting acceptance of uncertainty'. The women in this book were already grappling with uncertainty provoked by discrepancy between their own assessment of their risk and that of their professional carers. Their stories are important because they bring this discrepancy into the daylight, and demand that there be an egalitarian and informed debate between all those with a stake in the outcome of their pregnancies. They challenged the clearly indefensible notion that health professionals may be more committed to achieving a positive outcome to pregnancy than mothers are (Jordan and Murphy 2009: 196). They resisted the urge on the part of staff to treat them like children lacking in common sense, intellectual maturity and moral responsibility and took ownership of their pregnancies in the spirit of the National Health Service choice agenda.

How is acceptance of uncertainty and rediscovery of woman-centred care to be achieved? More can be gained through partnership than by any group standing alone. The strongest and the most logical partnership is likely to be between women and midwives. If women can trust midwives to be their advocates and to practise a midwifery rooted in observation and understanding of normal birth, women, midwives and normal birth will thrive. If midwives can demonstrate their confidence in midwifery knowledge and in women's innate capacity to give birth, they will increase women's faith in themselves and in midwifery. Midwives may fear handing power to women if they advocate for all the choices that women want to make, but in the world of 'realpolitik', they are more likely to retain power themselves if they support the power of maternity service consumers. While there may be professional groups who do not see that increasing the power of patients is in the best interests of patients, ideologically this is not a position that midwifery can support. For better or worse, if midwifery is to survive, it has to throw in its hand with women.

The maternity service, like the NHS overall, is a political arena. Its ideology, policies, funding and power derive from politics. Weston (2005) has argued that it is not possible to avoid politics if childbirth is to be liberated:

> Silence is complicity and doing nothing for change is passively supporting the status quo.

Midwives cannot choose to be apolitical. The continuance of their profession will depend on reframing society's ambivalence towards pregnancy, its tendency to fear pregnancy rather than to celebrate it, its focus on tests and interventions rather than on the mother's happiness and well-being. Midwifery must tackle this ambivalence and play a major part in creating communities dedicated from pregnancy onwards to supporting sensitive and responsive parenting.

We are in an era of economic re-evaluation; the average uncomplicated vaginal birth costs 68 per cent less in a home birth setting than in a hospital according to an American study (Anderson 1999) of sufficient quality to be included in the NHS Economic Evaluation Database (EED) (Fullerton *et al.* 2007). Although the NHS EED questioned whether the findings from this study could be generalized to other countries, it does not seem unreasonable to presume that straightforward vaginal birth is likely to be less costly in the UK as well as in America than caesarean section, and that home birth *may* be less expensive than hospital birth. From an economic viewpoint, therefore, this is a point in time when policy makers and health care managers may commit to shifting the balance of power away from experts in the biomedical model of care who have created a maternity service characterized by high rates of expensive interventions and towards those other experts, mothers and midwives, whose understandings have been put into the shade for the last 40 years. Government rhetoric already supports such a shift, and women's organizations are finding weapons to hand in documents such as *Maternity Matters* (2007).

The women in this book took the implied direction of travel of government and health service policy. They were independent and responsible health care consumers; they sought information from a variety of sources, including both professionals and their peer group – women who had already had babies; they made their own behavioural choices and were not prepared to delegate these to health professionals; they knew what they wanted to achieve and sought out people with the skills to help them achieve it; they were optimistic about pregnancy and recognized that they had personal strengths that would enable them to give birth and parent successfully. Despite the difficulties they encountered, they pursued their chosen course because they believed that the quality of the experience of birth and early parenting is critical for the development of healthy parents, children, families and society. They would have applauded Luke Zander (cited in Nolan 2009: 44) when he insisted at a conference more than 25 years ago that if we can get birth right, we can get society right.

References

Anderson B. (2010) Shock, horror: America places its own interests first. *The International Independent*, 29 March, p. 27.

Anderson R. (1999) The cost-effectiveness of home birth. *Journal of Nurse-Midwifery*, 44(1):30–5.

Department of Health (2004) The national service framework for children, young people and maternity services: standard 11. London: DH.

Department of Health (2007) *Maternity Matters: Choice, access and continuity of care in a safe service*. London: DH.

Dodwell M. (2009) (BirthChoiceUK) Personal communication.

Enkin M., Glouberman S., Groff P., Jadad A. and Stern A. (2006) Beyond evidence: the complexity of maternity care. *Birth*, 33(4):265–9.

Flint C. (1986) *Sensitive Midwifery*. London: Butterworth Heinemann.

Foucault M. (2001) *Madness and Civilization*. London: Routledge.

Fullerton T., Navarro A. M. and Young S. H. (2007) Outcomes of planned home birth: an integrative review. Database of Abstracts of Reviews of Effects (DARE), available online at www.crd.york.ac.uk/CRDWeb/ShowRecord.asp?ID=12007002365 (accessed 27 April 2010).

Gilbert P. (2009) *The Compassionate Mind*. Oakland, California: New Harbinger Publications.

Goodman P., Mackey M. C. and Tavakoli A. S. (2004) Factors related to childbirth satisfaction. *Journal of Advanced Nursing*, 46(2):212–9.

Gould D. (2004) Trust me, I am a midwife. *British Journal of Midwifery*, 12(1):44.

Green J. (1998) *Great Expectations: a prospective study of women's expectations and experiences of childbirth*. Oxford: Butterworth Heinemann.

Hay D. F., Pawlby S. and Angold, A. (2003) Pathways to violence in the children of mothers who were depressed postpartum. *Developmental Psychology*, 39:1083–94.

Heron J., O'Connor T., Evans J., Golding J. and Glover V. (2004) The course of anxiety and depression through pregnancy and the postpartum in a community sample. *Journal of Affective Disorders*, 80(1):65–73.

Hindley C. and Thomson A. M. (2005) The rhetoric of informed choice: perspectives from midwives on intrapartum fetal heart rate monitoring. *Health Expectations*, 8:306–14.

Houghton G., Bedwell C., Forsey M., Baker L., Lavender T. (2008) Factors influencing choice in birth place: an exploration of the views of women, their partners and professionals. *Evidence-Based Midwifery*, June, available online at www.rcm.org.uk (accessed 17 March 2010).

Hunter B., Berg M., Lundgren I., Ólafsdóttir O. and Kirkham M. (2008) Relationships: the hidden threads in the tapestry of maternity care. *Midwifery*, 24:132–7.

Jordan R. G. and Murphy P. Aikins (2009) Risk assessment and risk distortion: finding the balance. *Journal of Midwifery and Women's Health*, 54(3):191–200.

Kirkham M., Stapleton H., Curtis P. and Thomas G. (2002) Stereotyping as a professional defence mechanism. *British Journal of Midwifery*, 10(9):549–52.

Martin C. J. H. (2007) 'Obedience: would you do as I say?' *MIDIRS Midwifery Digest*, 17(1):7–13.

Maternity Care Working Party (National Childbirth Trust/Royal College of Midwives/

Royal College of Obstetricians and Gynaecologists) (2007) Making normal birth a reality. London: NCT/RCM/RCOG.

Midwives Information and Resource Service (2008) *Where will you have your baby? Informed Choice Leaflet 10*. Bristol: MIDIRS in collaboration with the Centre for Reviews and Dissemination.

Murray L. and Cooper P. J. (1996) The impact of postpartum depression on child development. *International Review of Psychiatry*, 8:55.

Murray L., Sinclair D. and Cooper P. (1999) The socioemotional development of 5-year-old children of postnatally depressed mothers. *Journal of Child Psychology and Psychiatry and Allied Disciplines*, 40:1259–1271.

Nolan M. (2009) Childbirth education: politics, equality and relevance. In: Walsh D. and Downe S. (eds) *Essential Midwifery Practice: intrapartum care*, Oxford: Blackwell Publishing: 31–44.

Pilley Edwards N. (2005) *Birthing Autonomy: Women's experiences of planning home births*. London: Routledge.

Robinson J. (2002) Scapegoats. *British Journal of Midwifery*, 10(5):278.

Stapleton H., Kirkham M., Thomas G. and Curtis P. (2002) Midwives in the middle: balance and vulnerability. *British Journal of Midwifery*, 10(10):607–11.

Stewart M. (2001) Whose evidence counts? An exploration of health professionals' perceptions of evidence-based practice, focusing in the maternity services. *Midwifery*, 17:279–88.

Talge N. M., Neal C. and Glover V. (2007) Antenatal maternal stress and long-term effects on child neurodevelopment: how and why? *Journal of Child Psychology and Psychiatry*, 48(3–4):245–61.

Uvnäs Moberg K. (2003) *The Oxytocin Factor*. US: Da Capo Press.

Viisainen K. (2001) Negotiating control and meaning: home birth as a self-constructed choice in Finland. *Social Science and Medicine*, 52:1109–1121.

Walsh D. (2006) Subverting the assembly line: childbirth in a free-standing birth centre. *Social Science and Medicine*, 62(6):1330–40.

Weston R. Sharples (2005) Liberating childbirth. *AIMS Journal*, 17(3), available online at www.aims.org.uk/Journal/Vol17No3/liberatingChildbirth.htm (accessed 2 April 2010).

Websites

BirthChoiceUK: www.birthchoiceuk.com/BirthChoiceUKFrame.htm? www.birthchoice uk.com/HomeBirthRates.htm (accessed 18 April 2010).

Home Birth Reference Site: www.homebirth.org.uk/ (accessed 18 April 2010).

Weston R. Sharples (2005) Liberating childbirth: www.aims.org.uk/Journal/Vol17No3/ liberatingChildbirth.htm (accessed 2 April 2010).

Conclusion

A Manifesto

1 Every woman's choice deserves respect and the effort to explore and understand it.
2 The big picture from the woman's standpoint may look very different from that of the maternity service.
3 The woman is the expert on her own body. The midwife is the expert on women's bodies.
4 The woman's emotional state in pregnancy – proud and confident or unsure and dependent – will affect her relationship with her baby.
5 Pregnancy is part of a continuum that ends, if it ends at all, with the coming of age of a new citizen.
6 Policy and protocol, pursued without regard for the individual, can easily turn into bullying and coercion.
7 It is never justified for a woman to leave a maternity consultation with her self-esteem lower than it was before.
8 Women value and have the highest respect for basic midwifery skills.
9 If, in practice, informed choice has limitations, it would be honest to modify the rhetoric of choice.
10 The current gulf between rhetoric and women's experience of the maternity service threatens the service and midwifery in particular.

Index

Note: page numbers in **bold** refer to figures and tables.